Mona Sedrak

Understanding the Role of Achievement Motivation in Medical Education

Mona Sedrak

Understanding the Role of Achievement Motivation in Medical Education

VDM Verlag Dr. Müller

Impressum/Imprint (nur für Deutschland/ only for Germany)
Bibliografische Information der Deutschen Nationalbibliothek: Die Deutsche Nationalbibliothek verzeichnet diese Publikation in der Deutschen Nationalbibliografie; detaillierte bibliografische Daten sind im Internet über http://dnb.d-nb.de abrufbar.

Alle in diesem Buch genannten Marken und Produktnamen unterliegen warenzeichen-, marken- oder patentrechtlichem Schutz bzw. sind Warenzeichen oder eingetragene Warenzeichen der jeweiligen Inhaber. Die Wiedergabe von Marken, Produktnamen, Gebrauchsnamen, Handelsnamen, Warenbezeichnungen u.s.w. in diesem Werk berechtigt auch ohne besondere Kennzeichnung nicht zu der Annahme, dass solche Namen im Sinne der Warenzeichen- und Markenschutzgesetzgebung als frei zu betrachten wären und daher von jedermann benutzt werden dürften.

Coverbild: www.ingimage.com

Verlag: VDM Verlag Dr. Müller GmbH & Co. KG
Dudweiler Landstr. 99, 66123 Saarbrücken, Deutschland
Telefon +49 681 9100-698, Telefax +49 681 9100-988
Email: info@vdm-verlag.de
Zugl.: Minneapolis, MN, Walden University, Diss., 2003

Herstellung in Deutschland:
Schaltungsdienst Lange o.H.G., Berlin
Books on Demand GmbH, Norderstedt
Reha GmbH, Saarbrücken
Amazon Distribution GmbH, Leipzig
ISBN: 978-3-8364-8252-3

Imprint (only for USA, GB)
Bibliographic information published by the Deutsche Nationalbibliothek: The Deutsche Nationalbibliothek lists this publication in the Deutsche Nationalbibliografie; detailed bibliographic data are available in the Internet at http://dnb.d-nb.de.

Any brand names and product names mentioned in this book are subject to trademark, brand or patent protection and are trademarks or registered trademarks of their respective holders. The use of brand names, product names, common names, trade names, product descriptions etc. even without a particular marking in this works is in no way to be construed to mean that such names may be regarded as unrestricted in respect of trademark and brand protection legislation and could thus be used by anyone.

Cover image: www.ingimage.com

Publisher: VDM Verlag Dr. Müller GmbH & Co. KG
Dudweiler Landstr. 99, 66123 Saarbrücken, Germany
Phone +49 681 9100-698, Fax +49 681 9100-988
Email: info@vdm-publishing.com

Printed in the U.S.A.
Printed in the U.K. by (see last page)
ISBN: 978-3-8364-8252-3

Copyright © 2011 by the author and VDM Verlag Dr. Müller GmbH & Co. KG and licensors
All rights reserved. Saarbrücken 2011

TABLE OF CONTENTS

Page

CHAPTER 1: INTRODUCTION TO THE STUDY 1
Introduction 1
Problem Statement 3
Purpose 4
Research Questions 5
Research Design and Scope 5
Theoretical Framework 6
Significance of the Study 8
Definitions 8
Assumptions and Limitations 10
Summary 11

CHAPTER 2: REVIEW OF THE LITERATURE 13
Introduction 13
Achievement Motivation 14
The Achievement Goal Theory 16
Intrinsic Motivation and Achievement Goals 19
Defining Goal Orientation 21
A Trichotomous Approach 23
Classroom Implications 26
A Developmental Perspective 28
Summary 32

CHAPTER 3: METHODOLOGY AND RESEARCH DESIGN 34
Introduction 34
Research Design 34
Research Questions and Statistical Hypotheses 35
Population 36
Sample 37
Variables 37
Instrumentation 38
Procedures for Data Collection 40
Data Analysis 41
Characteristics of the Data 41
Statistical Measures 42
Social Change 43
Summary 43

CHAPTER 4: RESULTS 45
Introduction 45
Description of the Sample 46

Description of the Data Gathered From the Instrument 48
Testing the Research Hypotheses 49
Research Hypotheses 1 and 2 49
Research Hypothesis 3 52
Summary 55

CHAPTER 5: SUMMARY, CONCLUSIONS, AND RECOMENDATIONS 57
Summary of Research Finding 57
Conclusions from the Hypotheses 59
Research Hypotheses 1 and 2 59
Research Hypothesis 3 62
Younger Cohort and Middle Cohort 62
Older Cohort 64
Revised Age Categories 64
Delineation of the Age Cohorts 66
Implications for Social Change 68
Recommendations 70

REFERENCES 73

APPENDIX A: The Goals Inventory 81

APPENDIX B: Invitation to Programs 82

APPENDIX C: Program Informational Form 84

APPENDIX D: Instructions for Site Coordinators 85

APPENDIX E: Invitation to Participate/Consent Statement 87

APPENDIX F: Permission to Use Instrument 89

CHAPTER 1

INTRODUCTION TO THE STUDY

Introduction

Vago (1999) commented, "Everywhere change has become central to people's awareness and there is a commitment to change that is irreversible, irresistible, and irrevocable" (p. 4). In no institution is societal change more evident than in the medical community. In the United States, approximately 71.7 million people are expected to be 55 years or older by 2010, 15.4 million people more than this demographic cohort represented in 2000 (Berman, 2001). Advances in medical technology are permitting an increasing number of health care problems to be treated, thereby increasing life expectancies. These advances, linked with an aging population, have generated an increased demand for health services and an increase in health care spending (Berman, 2001; Hecker, 2001).

Currently, there is a nationwide trend to stem the rapid growth of spending on health care by medical insurers and the government (Berman, 2001; Hecker, 2001). In response to this effort, the utilization of physician assistants (PAs) in the hospital and clinic setting has increased as PAs assume some duties formerly performed by more highly paid health care workers. Remarkably, the Department of Labor has projected a 48 % increase in the number of physician assistant jobs between 1998 and 2008 (Association of Physician Assistant Programs, 2001, p. 3).

Vago (1999) argued that institutions of higher education have a responsibility to respond to social change by adequately preparing students to join the workforce. In response to increasing market demands for physician assistants, there has been a rapid proliferation of PA educational programs nationwide (Simon, Link, & Miko, 2002). However, these programs are experiencing demographic changes in their enrollment patterns that may affect their ability to fully respond to the projected market demands of the future.

In the *18th Annual Report on Physician Assistant Educational Programs in the United States, 2001-2002*, Simon et al. (2002) discussed the demographics of both the applicants and enrolled students in PA programs nationwide. Of particular interest was the increase of enrollees less than 24 years of age. For the 2001-2002 academic year the proportion of enrollees less than 24 years of age increased to 27.4 % from a pattern of decrease through 1995 (p. 9). Although initially demonstrating a pattern of decrease from 1983 to 1992, enrollment of students between the ages of 24 and 29 has gradually increased to the current level of 39.7 %. Furthermore, enrollment of students over 29 years of age had systematically increased from 1983 to 1992 and then decreased to the current level of 32.8 % (p.9). Simon et al. (2002) noted that this is the 4th year since 1986 that the percentage of students over 29 years of age was less than the 24 to 29 year old group. Furthermore, these researchers reported that attrition was highest for students 20 to 23 years of age. Of those students who withdrew from their program of study during the 2001-2002 academic year, 47.8 % reported academic reasons.

Although many factors influence academic performance, the achievement motivation literature suggests that success may depend on the achievement goals that students adopt within the educational setting and the consequences of those goals on educational outcomes (Covington, 2000; Dweck, 1986, Harackiewicz, Barron, & Elliot, 1998; Nicholls 1984). Burley, Turner, and Vitulli (1999) noted, at the college level, the tendency to pursue one motivational goal more than another may be influenced by student age.

Numerous studies have investigated the relationship between achievement goal orientation and academic success at the collegiate level (Harackiewicz et al., 1998; Harackiewicz, Barron, Tauer, Carter, & Elliot, 2000; Hayamizu & Weiner, 1991; Miller, Brehens, Greene, & Newman, 1993; Roedal & Schraw, 1995; Schraw, Horn, Thorndike-Christ, & Bruning, 1995; Shields, 1993); however, a recent review of the literature by this researcher identified only one study (Burley et al., 1999) that specifically addressed achievement goal orientation and student age. Due to the limited research available that specifically addresses achievement goal orientation and student age at the college level, a gap in the literature existed.

Problem Statement

In the *18th Annual Report on Physician Assistant Educational Programs in the United States, 2001-2002,* Simon et al. (2002) noted an increased enrollment of younger students in the United States. This report documented higher attrition rates for this younger cohort in comparison to their older peers. While many factors may influence academic performance, success may depend on the motivational goals that students pursue in the educational context (Covington, 2000; Dweck, 1986; Harackiewicz et al., 1998; Nicholls, 1984). Researchers have confirmed important differences in the motivational attitudes of younger and older students that impact their motivational goals and thus their academic performance (Burley et al., 1999; Werring, 1987; Wolfgang & Dowling, 1981).

Ames (1992) suggested that motivation and learning are facilitated by certain classroom characteristics such as the types of academic tasks students are assigned, classroom authority, and the criteria used for evaluation and recognition. Understanding the relationship between achievement goal orientation and student age may encourage educators to tailor future courses and curricula to foster an atmosphere that better facilitates motivation and learning in their student population. Furthermore, educators may be able to identify students at risk for academic hardship, develop intervention strategies, and effectively administer those strategies thereby improving student learning and lowering attrition rates. Given the rising demand for qualified PAs to meet the needs of an aging public and an overwhelmed health care system (Berman, 2001; Hecker, 2001), PA educators must respond by developing a clearer understanding of the motivational goals of this increasingly younger student population and making the necessary adjustments to improve attrition rate.

Purpose

The relationship between achievement goal orientation and academic performance has been studied at the collegiate level since the early 1990s (Harackiewicz et al., 1998, 2000; Hayamizu & Weiner, 1991; Miller et al., 1993; Roedal & Schraw, 1995; Schraw et al., 1995). A review of the literature by this researcher, however, identified only one study that investigated the relationship between student age and achievement goal orientation at the collegiate level (Burley et al., 1999). Building on Dweck (1986) and Nicholl's (1984) theory of achievement motivation, the primary purpose of the study was to address this gap in the literature by examining the relationship between achievement goal orientation and student age in physician assistant students.

Research Questions

1. What is the nature of the relationship between achievement goal orientation and student age?
2. What is the difference in the achievement goals students endorse across the age cohorts?

Research Design and Scope

To study the relationship between achievement goal orientation and student age at the college level, this study employed a nonexperimental quantitative design. Sampling first-year physician assistant students enrolled in baccalaureate programs in the United States, the study utilized the *Goals Inventory*, a Likert scale instrument, to determine the achievement goal orientation of students. Students were also asked to self-report their age.

For the purpose of this study, the participant age data were disaggregated and grouped into three categories based on the trends in student demographics and attrition rates as reported by Simon et al. (2002). Participants who were less than 24 years of age were grouped into the "younger cohort" category while participants who were between the ages of 24 to 29 were grouped into a "middle cohort" category. Finally, participants older than 29 years of age were grouped into the "older cohort" category.

To describe the nature of the relationship between achievement goal orientation and student age, the Spearman test and analysis of variance (ANOVA) were employed. To make decisions about whether there was a relationship between two or more variables, chi-square analysis was employed.

Exploring the variable of student age as it relates to achievement goal orientation in PA students is of particular importance given the trends in student age and attrition demographics noted by Simon et al. (2002). In the event that these trends continue, educators and administrators who have traditionally experienced an older student population must prepare to meet the challenge of educating a younger student population.

Theoretical Framework

Achievement goal theory was first introduced in the late 1970s and early 1980s by Carol Dweck (1986), John Nicholls (1984), and others (Ames & Ames, 1984; Dweck & Bempechat, 1983; Maehr & Nicholls, 1980; Nicholls, 1979, 1984). In a number of studies, achievement goal theorists identified two distinct types of achievement goal orientations: mastery goals and performance goals (Ames, 1992; Meece, Blumenfeld, & Hoyle, 1988; Nicholls, Patashick, Cheung, Thorkildsen, & Lauer, 1989). Each orientation represents a different way of thinking about competence and creates a framework for how individuals approach, experience, and react to achievement situations (Ames & Archer, 1988; Dweck & Leggett, 1988; Nicholls, 1984).

Through the use of experimental and quasi-experimental research designs, investigators confirmed a direct association between achievement goal orientation and academic outcomes (Meece & Holt, 1993; Pokay & Blumenfeld, 1990). The early research posited that mastery goals were adaptive while performance goals were maladaptive (Pintrich & De Groot, 1990; Pintrich & Garcia, 1991; Pintrich, Roser, & De Groot, 1994; Pintrich & Schrauben, 1992; Wolters, Yu, & Pintrich, 1996). However, as discussed in chapter 2, the debate regarding conflicting theoretical considerations and empirical results continues and suggests that a performance goal orientation might not always show a negative relation with motivation, cognition, and performance (Harackiewciz et al., 1998, 2000; Rawsthorne & Elliot, 1999; Pintrich, 2000).

Much of the research in the area of achievement goal orientation has focused on elementary and secondary school students. It was not until the early 1990s that studies began to address achievement goal orientation and academic success at the collegiate level (Harackiewciz et al., 1998, 2000; Hayamizu & Weiner, 1991; Miller et al., 1993; Roedal & Schraw, 1995; Schraw et al., 1995; Shields, 1993). Collegiate populations differ from elementary and secondary school populations in important ways. First, in collegiate populations there exists a heterogeneous population of older and younger students. Researchers contend that important differences exist in the motivational attitudes of older and younger students that may impact their achievement goal orientation and hence their academic performance (Burley et al., 1999; Werring, 1987; Wolfgang & Dowling, 1981).

Also, as students progress through the educational system, increasing demands are placed on them (Anderman, Austin, & Johnson, 2002). Whereas elementary schools do not often focus on students' abilities in comparison to other students, at the junior high school and high school level there is an increasing emphasis on ability, performance, and grades (Anderman et al., 2002). At the college level, this translates into a highly competitive environment, which, according to some researchers (Anderman et al., 2002; Harackiewicz et al., 1998), may influence achievement goal orientation.

Although researchers have explored the relationship between academic performance and achievement goal orientation in college students (Harackiewicz et al., 1998, 2000; Hayamizu & Weiner, 1991; Miller et al., 1993; Roedal & Schraw, 1995;

Schraw et al., 1995; Shields, 1993), a review of the literature identified only one study that investigated the relationship between student age and achievement goal orientation at the college level (Burley et al., 1999). Burley et al. (1999) defined "younger" as students 17 to 24 years of age and "older" as students 25 years of age and older. These researchers concluded that older students were more likely to be mastery goal oriented than their younger peers. However, the authors suggested additional research of the study to confirm these findings.

Significance of the Study

There is considerable evidence that achievement motivation and learning are facilitated in certain classroom environments (Ames, 1992; Blumenfeld, 1992; Meece et al., 1988). Forming a clearer understanding of the relationship between achievement goal orientation and student age at the college level may impact future curricular development as educators tailor courses and curricula to foster an atmosphere that better facilitates motivation and learning in their student population. Furthermore, educators may also be able to identify students at risk for academic hardships and develop effective intervention strategies (Eppler & Harju, 1997). Combined, these efforts may positively impact student retention rates, thereby lowering attrition. This is of particular importance to PA educators, given the student age and attrition trends of enrolling PA students noted by Simon et al. (2002) as well as the increased demand for PAs in the health care market (Hecker, 2001).

Definition of Terms

The following conceptual definitions are provided to clarify the meanings of the terms utilized in the proposed study:

Achievement goal orientation: Goal orientation represents an integrated pattern of beliefs that lead to different ways of approaching, engaging in, and responding to achievement situations (Ames, 1992).

Adaptive motivational patterns: Adaptive motivational patterns are those that promote the establishment, maintenance, and attainment of personally challenging and personally valued achievement goals (Dweck, 1986).

Age: For the purposes of data analyses, the participants who were less than 24 years of age were grouped into the "younger cohort" category while the participants who were between the ages of 24 to 29 were grouped into a "middle cohort" category. The participants older than 29 years of age were grouped into the "older cohort" category. These categories were formed based on trends in student demographics and attrition rates as reported by Simon et al. (2002).

Drives: A drive is an internal state, need, or condition that impels individuals toward action (Covington, 2000).

Goals: Goals represent the very specific purposes that individuals are striving for in a specific setting (Wolters et al., 1996).

Intrinsic motivation: Intrinsic motivation is interest in and the enjoyment of an activity for its own sake (Rawsthorne & Elliot, 1999).

Maladaptive motivational patterns: Maladaptive motivational patterns are those that are associated with a failure to establish reasonable, valued goals, and to maintain effective striving toward those goals (Dweck, 1986).

Metacogniton: Metacognition refers both to the explicit knowledge individuals have about their cognitive resources and to the deliberate self-regulation they can exercise when applying this knowledge (Bouffard, Boisvert, Vezeau, & Larouche, 1995).

Nontraditional students: As defined by Eppler and Harju (1997), nontraditional students are older students, between the ages of 22-53, who had taken a year or more away from college and pursued other career and family goals before continuing with their studies.

Physician assistants: Physician assistants are health professionals licensed or credentialed to practice medicine with physician supervision (American Academy of Physician Assistants, 1998).

Physician assistant student: A physician assistant student is an individual enrolled in a physician assistant program accredited by the Accreditation Review Commission on Education for Physician Assistants (American Academy of Physician Assistants, 1998).

Self-regulated learning: Self-regulated learning is how students select, organize, or create an advantageous learning environment for themselves and how they plan and control the form and amount of their own instruction (Zimmerman, 1990).

Traditional students: As defined by Eppler and Harju (1997), traditional students are younger students, less than 22 years of age, who have been enrolled continuously in school since high school graduation.

Assumptions and Limitations

There were three assumptions of the study: (a) students accurately report their age; (b) students would answer the *Goals Inventory* in a manner that accurately represents their academic experiences; and (c) although the *Goals Inventory* is a previously validated instrument (Roedel, Schraw, & Plake, 1994), it is only one measure of achievement goal orientation. Although there are other instruments such as the *Personality Research Form* and *the Motivated Strategies for Learning Questionnaire* that test for goal orientation, the *Goals Inventory* was chosen for the following reasons. First, the *Goals Inventory* is a complete instrument, rather than a subset of another instrument, that specifically tests for mastery goals and performance goals rather than a combination of mastery/performance goals and approach/avoidance goals (Barron & Harackiewcz, 2001; Pintrich, 2000). Second, the *Goals Inventory* provides separate scores for mastery goals and performance goals rather than treating these variables as if they were opposite endpoints of a single, continuous dimension (Eison, 1981; Eppler & Harju, 1997).

There were two limitations of the study. First, the study examined a targeted sample of physician assistant students. For this reason it was expected that the participants of the study would not be representative of all physician assistant students. Second, although gender, socioeconomic status, culture, ethnicity, previous academic experience, and previous health care experience may impact motivation, the study did not investigate these variables.

Summary

Academic success at the college and university level is typically defined in terms of performance where grades are utilized as an indicator of performance (Harackiewicz et al., 1998). Achievement motivation theorists contend that success may depend on the achievement goals that students adopt within the educational setting and the consequences of those goals on educational outcomes (Covington, 2000; Dweck, 1986; Harackiewicz et al., 1998; Nicholls, 1984). While the concept of achievement goal orientation has been discussed in scientific psychology for over a century (Elliot &

Harackiewicz, 1996), there continues to be debate regarding the adaptive and maladaptive properties of mastery goals and performance goals.

In contemporary achievement motivation literature, achievement goal theory continues to be the most influential and accepted theory in differentiating competence-based strivings (Elliot & Harackiewicz, 1996; Wolters, 1998). Extending Dweck (1986) and Nicholl's (1984) achievement goal theory to the collegiate level, the study examined the relationship between achievement goal orientation and student age in physician assistant students by identifying the differences in the achievement goals that students endorse across the age cohorts.

This chapter provided a brief introduction to achievement motivation and developed the purpose of the study and research questions, scope, theoretical framework, significance, assumptions, and limitations. Chapter 2 is a review of the literature on achievement goal theory and its relationship to academic performance. Chapter 3 outlines the research design of the study and discusses the procedures that were used in the collection, management, and analyses of the data.

CHAPTER 2

REVIEW OF THE LITERATURE

Introduction

This chapter presents the theoretical literature on achievement motivation that served as the foundation for the study. The chapter begins with a historical review of the experimental and quasi-experimental research that examines the foundation and development of achievement goal theory from its earliest form in the 1950s through the present. The next section explores the complex aspects of achievement goal theory, introducing and examining the primary orientations of mastery goal orientation and performance goal orientation and their impact on academic achievement and intrinsic motivation. Also, the chapter examines the on-going debate in the achievement motivation literature regarding the adaptive and maladaptive qualities of performance goals. Finally, the chapter examines the classroom implications of achievement goal theory and concludes with a developmental perspective of achievement goals.

The concept of motivation stands at the center of the educational enterprise (Ames, 1992; Elliot & Harackiewicz, 1996; Eppler & Harju, 1997; Roedel & Schraw, 1995; Schraw et al., 1995). Contemporary research on achievement motivation is based largely on an analysis of the achievement goals of individuals that are defined as the purpose of or reason for competence-relevant activity (Ames, 1992; Maehr, 1989). A number of researchers have contrasted different types of achievement goals and examined the effects of these goals on a variety of cognitive, affective, and behavioral outcomes (Ames, 1992; Dweck, 1986; Maehr, 1989; Nicholls, 1984).

In the process of researching the literature, a number of databases were utilized. To search the psychological literature the following databases were utilized: PsychInfo and PsychArticles. To search the sociological literature, Sociological Abstracts was utilized. To search the educational literature, ERIC and Educational Abstracts were utilized. Finally, to search the medical literature, Medline and CINAHL were used. The following keywords guided the search: motivation, achievement motivation, achievement goals, need achievement theory, intrinsic motivation, academic performance, and student age. A synthesis of the research relevant to the study is offered in the following review of the literature.

Achievement Motivation

Vander Zanden (1987) defined motivation as "those inner states and processes that prompt, direct, and sustain activity" (p. 300). Dweck (1986) stated that motivational processes are responsible for the "acquisition, transfer, and use of knowledge and skills" (p.1040). Over the past century, two very different conceptions of achievement motivation have emerged: motives as drives and motives as goals (Covington, 2000).

The first conceptualization of achievement motivation viewed motivation as a drive where needs were thought to reside largely within the individual. These notions evolved from earlier theories of motivation that emphasized the satisfaction of such basic needs as hunger and thirst (Vander Zanden, 1987). However, there are limitations to applying a strictly physiological approach to explaining human behavior and researchers eventually broadened their focus to include learned drives such as the need for social approval, power, and achievement.

Lewin and his colleagues (Lewin, Dembo, Festinger, & Sears, 1944) first discussed achievement motivation as a learned drive in the 1940s. These researchers identified two independent motivational orientations: the desire for success and the desire to avoid failure. Building on the work of Lewin et al. (1944), McClelland (1951) affirmed these two distinctions of achievement motivation. Drawing on the work of Lewin et al. (1944) and McClelland (1951), Atkinson (1957) formulated the "need achievement theory" that was structured on a mathematical framework and reaffirmed the two motivational dispositions.

These two motivational dispositions, termed approach and avoidance, were mainly characterized in emotional terms. For instance, striving for success and anticipating winning was said to encourage success-oriented individuals, while a capacity for experiencing shame was said to drive failure-oriented individuals to avoid situations in which they anticipated failure. The balance or imbalance between these two dispositions were said to determine the intensity, quality, and direction of achievement behaviors (Covington, 2000). It was this difference in emotional reactions between pride or shame that was thought to answer the question of why some individuals approach learning with enthusiasm while others, anticipating failure, avoid challenging situations (Middleton & Midgley, 1997).

In the early 1970s, however, a dramatic change took place in the study of motivation (Covington, 2000; Dweck, 1986). This change resulted in "a coherent, replicable, and educationally relevant body of findings and a clearer understanding of motivational phenomena" (Dweck, 1986, p. 1040). Dweck (1986) commented that it was during this time that emphasis shifted to a social-cognitive approach and away from "external contingencies" and "global internal states" (p. 1040). This shift allowed researchers to characterize adaptive and maladaptive patterns, explain these patterns in terms of specific underlying processes, and develop a conceptual framework for intervention (Dweck, 1986, p. 1040).

By the late 1970s and early 1980s, Carol Dweck, John Nicholls, and others (Dweck & Bempechat, 1983; Maher, 1989; Maehr & Nicholls, 1980; Nicholls, 1979, 1984) introduced an achievement goal approach to achievement motivation theory and defined achievement goals as the reason for, or purpose of, competence relevant activity. These theorists postulated a casual relationship between the goal orientation of a student and their behavioral responses in an academic setting (Dweck, 1986; Nicholls, 1984).

The Achievement Goal Theory

In the late 1980s, achievement goal theory became the predominant approach used in the analysis of achievement motivation. Initially, achievement goal theorists incorporated the approach-avoidance distinctions in their theoretical frameworks. Dweck and Elliot (1983) and Nicholls (1984) identified three types of achievement goals in their early work: a mastery or task involvement goal, which focused on the development of competence and task mastery (approach orientation); a performance or ego involvement goal, directed toward attaining favorable judgments of competence (also an approach orientation); and a performance or ego involvement goal aimed at avoiding unfavorable judgments of competence (an avoidance orientation). However, the concept of approach and avoidance as independent orientations received little theoretical and no empirical attention and therefore was soon abandoned (Covington, 2000; Dweck, 1986). Most theorists then shifted to a performance-mastery goal dichotomy while the approach-avoidance components collapsed into a unitary orientation (Elliot & Harackiewicz, 1996).

By the late 1980s and early 1990s, most contemporary achievement goal theorists began to structure their theories similar to the revised models of Dweck (1986) and Nicholls (1984) in two important ways. First, most theorists began to articulate two primary orientations toward competence (Elliot & Harackiewicz, 1996). Ames (1984) differentiated mastery and ability goals; Roberts (1992) studied mastery and competitive goals; and Deci and Ryan (1985) contrasted task and ego involvement. Ames and Archer (1988) and Ryan and Stiller (1991) later argued that each of these frameworks was conceptually similar and allowed for convergence in the form of a mastery goal (mastery, learning, and ego involvement) and a performance goal (performance, ability, ego involvement, and competitive) distinction. Second, all the aforementioned theorists either characterized mastery goals and performance goals as approach forms of motivation (Ames, 1992; Meece et al., 1988; Nicholls et al., 1989) or they failed to consider approach and avoidance as independent motivational tendencies within the performance goal orientation (Dweck, 1986; Meece et al., 1988).

Achievement goal theorists contend that the type of orientation adopted at the outset of an activity creates a framework for how individuals interpret and act on achievement relevant information and experience achievement settings (Elliot & Harackiewicz, 1996). Mastery goals are considered adaptive because they are related to positive educational outcomes such as long-term learning, the use of deep cognitive strategies, and the ability to relate material to prior knowledge (Anderman et al., 2002). Students with a "mastery" motivational pattern prefer moderately challenging tasks, are persistent, especially in the face of failure, and have a positive outlook on learning (Dweck, 1986).

A mastery goal orientation is characterized by a desire to acquire new skills and knowledge purely for the sake of learning. Students who adopt a mastery goal orientation focus on learning and mastery of the material for the purpose of improving competence rather than demonstrating their ability (Ames, 1992). Underlying the mastery goal orientation is the premise that effort is a means to success and that effort actually enhances ability (Eppler & Harju, 1997).

In both experimental and quasi-experimental studies a mastery goal orientation has been linked to the quality of students' cognitive engagement (Pintrich & Schrauben, 1992). For example, Graham and Golan (1991) found that students who adopted a mastery goal orientation were more likely to process the material being memorized at a deeper level. In correlational studies, Pintrich and his colleagues (Pintrich & De Groot, 1990; Pintrich & Gracia, 1991; Pintrich et al., 1994) showed that students who adopted a mastery orientation focused on learning the material by using cognitive strategies, such as elaboration and organization, which reflect deeper levels of cognitive processes. These relations hold for junior high, high school, and college students.

In contrast, the adoption of a performance goal orientation is hypothesized to produce a constellation of "helpless" motivational responses that produce a pattern of a preference for easy tasks and effort withdrawal in the face of failure (Elliot & Harackiewicz, 1996). Performance goals are also associated with lower levels of cognitive engagement such as the use of more surface level processing strategies like rehearsal instead of deeper processing strategies like elaboration (Nolen, 1988; Pintrich &

Schrauben, 1992; Wolters et al., 1996). This general orientation leads to a less adaptive attributional pattern such as attributing failure to a lack of ability and lower perceptions of competence and self-efficacy.

Research has shown that students who adopt this orientation tend to be focused on their performance relative to others and centered on their self-worth (Ames, 1992). As a result, students are likely to avoid challenge, especially when their perceptions of competence are low. However, even when perceptions of competence are high and individuals are confident they can perform well; performance-oriented students may sacrifice learning opportunities to look good in front of others (Harackiewicz et al., 1998).

Researchers such as Graham and Golan (1991), Elliot and Harackiewicz (1996), Pintrich and Schrauben (1992), Wolters et al. (1996) and others built on the original work of Dweck (1986) and Nicholls (1984). As demonstrated, these researchers, through experimental and nonexperimental studies, clarified the relationship between goal orientation and academic performance. Using this body of literature as a foundation, this study explored the additional variable of student age as it relates to students' endorsement of achievement goals.

Intrinsic Motivation and Achievement Goals

An important component of achievement goal theory often discussed in the literature is intrinsic motivation (Ames, 1992; Ryan, 1992). Intrinsic motivation is manifested in the enjoyment of, and interest in, an activity for its own sake (Ryan, 1992). In the academic setting, intrinsic motivation would be reflected in the active involvement of students in coursework, lectures, course material, and readings. Intrinsically motivated students enjoy learning and their questions to the instructor usually reflect the course subject matter rather than what specifically will be covered on an exam (Harackiewicz et al., 1998).

At the college and university level, intrinsic motivation is especially important to consider because the interests of students play a major role in determining the extent and direction of their continued studies (Harackiewicz et al., 1998). Because interest and performance both develop throughout the course of the educational process, it is possible that intrinsic interest can influence learning and performance (Harackiewicz et al., 1998; Rawsthorne & Elliot, 1999). For example, if a student becomes interested in the subject matter, he or she may devote more time and energy to the coursework and as a result, perform at a higher level. Thus, intrinsic motivation in a particular college course may not only influence performance in that course but also provide continued motivation beyond that course.

Most achievement goal theorists contend that mastery and performance goals produce distinct processes that have divergent consequences for intrinsic motivation (Rawsthorne & Elliot, 1999). Mastery goals are posited to encourage task absorption, support self-determination, and foster feelings of autonomy, all factors presumed to be facilitative of intrinsic factors (Butler, 1987; Dweck, 1986). In contrast, performance goals are portrayed as undermining intrinsic motivation by instilling perceptions of threat, disrupting task involvement, and eliciting anxiety and evaluative pressure (Elliot & Harackiewicz, 1996). Rawsthorne and Elliot (1999) argued that most theorists espouse a "main effect hypothesis," whereby individuals pursuing performance goals are expected to demonstrate lower levels of intrinsic motivation than their mastery oriented counterparts. Empirical investigations, however, have yielded mixed support for the main effect hypothesis.

Although a number of experimental studies have documented the undermining effects of performance goals on intrinsic motivation (Butler, 1987; Ryan, 1982; Ryan, Koestner, & Deci, 1991), other investigations have failed to provide supporting evidence (Butler, 1987; Harackiewicz & Elliot, 1993; Koestner, Zuckerman, & Koestner, 1989). Harackiewcz et al. (1998) contended that although performance goals may be more likely than mastery goals to foster an extrinsic orientation, they may not always have this effect. For example, performance goals may not impair intrinsic interest if students perceive themselves as competent. Also, Harackiewicz et al. (1998) stated that it is important to recognize the positive potential of performance goals. If individuals typically define competence in terms of ability, a performance goal orientation might make them more likely to think about or value their competence at an activity and, therefore, they may work harder and become more involved in their performance.

Defining Goal Orientations

Many studies over the past 20 years have utilized a goal orientation framework for studying achievement motivation. For mastery goals, the results have been fairly consistent; for performance goals the results have been less consistent (Anderman et al., 2002). In the literature, the contention that mastery goals are adaptive and performance goals are maladaptive is referred to as the mastery goal perspective (Ames, 1992). This theoretical perspective implies that individuals are more successful when they focus exclusively on mastery goals in their achievement pursuits.

There has been, however, some debate in the literature over the deleterious effect of performance goals. Several theorists have suggested that performance goals may in fact promote important achievement outcomes because such goals can help orient individuals toward competence (Eppler & Harju, 1997; Harackiewicz, Barron, Carter, Lehto, & Elliot, 1997; Harckiewicz & Elliot, 1993). Thus, a number of theorists have endorsed a multiple goal perspective in which adopting both types of achievement goals is considered most adaptive (Butler & Winne, 1995; Harackiewicz et al., 1998; Pintrich & Garcia, 1991).

The question, then, is why these two perspectives, that is, the mastery goal perspective and the multiple goal perspective, have emerged. The literature suggests that the strong conclusions about the negative effects of performance goals may have been premature (Harackiewicz et al., 1998; Rawsthorne & Elliot, 1999). Moreover, there are both conflicting theoretical considerations and empirical results that suggest that a performance goal orientation might not always show a negative relation with motivation, cognition, and performance. From a theoretical perspective, there is some debate whether mastery and performance goal orientations are orthogonal or negatively related to one another (Pintrich, 2000; Wolters et al., 1996). If they are orthogonal, and some research has shown that the goal orientations are independent dimensions, then it would be possible for students to show varying patterns of goal orientation (Dweck & Leggett, 1988).

Pintrich and Garcia (1991) suggested that there may be an advantage for students to be relatively high on both mastery and performance orientations. Butler and Winne (1995), based on quasi-experimental research, also argued that both mastery and performance orientations can be adopted by students and that this multiple goal orientation may provide students with important guides for interpreting feedback and regulating their learning. In Butler and Winne's (1995) model, a performance goal orientation can be useful to students as it would provide an additional external reference against which they can judge performance.

According to Barron and Harakiewicz (2001), in cases where researchers have used data analytic strategies such as multiple regression, structural equation modeling, or cluster analysis to test both perspectives, only a few studies have found that optimal achievement outcomes occur when students endorsed mastery goals but not performance goals (Meece & Holt, 1993; Pintrich & Garcia, 1991). Most of the research in this area found that optimal outcomes occur when both goals are pursued (Ainley, 1993; Bouffard et al., 1995; Elliot & Church, 1997; Harackiewicz et al., 1997, 2000; Pintrich, 2000; Wentzel, 1993).

In correlational studies, where students are typically surveyed in classroom settings and asked to indicate the extent to which they pursue each type of goal, researchers have consistently found that measures of mastery and performance goals were uncorrelated or even positively correlated (Harackiewicz et al., 1998). Given these findings and the possibility that individuals can and do pursue multiple goals, many researchers believe that it is critical to test the simultaneous effects of both mastery and performance goals as well as whether these goals interact (Harackiewicz et al., 1998).

A Trichotomous Approach

Offering an alternative explanation to the inconsistent research findings regarding performance goals, Anderman et al. (2002) contended that these inconsistencies occurred primarily because, prior to the mid-1990s, many researchers confounded the various types of performance goals (approach and avoidance). Elliot and Harackiewicz (1996) noted that most researchers focused exclusively on the "approach" components of mastery and performance goals but ignored the avoidance component and proposed that the conventional mastery/performance goal dictomy be expanded to incorporate approach and avoidance components within the performance goal orientation. Similar to the trichotomous model initially introduced by achievement goal theorists in the early 1980s and abandoned shortly there after (Dweck & Elliot, 1983; Nicholls, 1984), the model introduced by Elliot and Harackiewicz (1996) identified three goal orientations: mastery, performance-approach, and performance-avoidance.

This framework is process-oriented in nature. Here the approach and avoidance components exert differential effects on achievement behavior by activating divergent sets of motivational processes (Elliot & Harackiewicz, 1996). In this model, performance-approach and mastery orientations both represent approach orientations and are grounded in self-regulation according to potential positive outcomes. In contrast, the performance-avoidance goal orientation is conceptualized as an avoidance orientation grounded in self- regulation according to potential negative outcomes. This form of regulation evokes a self-protective process that interferes with optimal task engagement and leads to a helpless set of motivational responses (Elliot & Harackiewicz, 1996).

In this trichotomous goal theory perspective, an important distinction has been made between performance-approach and performance-avoidance goals (Elliot & Church, 1997; Middleton & Midgley, 1997; Skaalvik, 1997). Although in early research mastery goals were linked to adaptive outcomes and performance goals to maladaptive outcomes, Pintrich (2000) argued that, in this trichotomous approach, there might be situations where performance goals may not be maladaptive. Harackiewicz and Elliot (1993) and their colleagues (Elliot & Church, 1997; Elliot & Harackiewicz, 1996; Harackiewicz et al., 1997, 1998) showed that performance goals can result in better performance, whereas mastery goals are linked to more intrinsic interest in the task. In both correlational and experimental research, where mastery, performance-approach, and performance-avoidance goals are compared, maladaptive patterns of intrinsic motivation and actual performance occurred only in the performance-avoidance group (Elliot & Church, 1997; Elliot & Harackiewicz, 1996; Harackiewicz et al., 1998; Pintrich, 2000). In essence, this conceptualization is an integration of the classic and the contemporary approaches to achievement motivation.

In a performance-approach or mastery-approach orientation, individuals perceive the achievement setting as a challenge; this generates excitement and encourages a cognitive and affective investment. This orients the individual towards a success-relevant and mastery-relevant information process hypothesized to facilitate intrinsic motivation (Elliot & Harackiewicz, 1996; Pintrich, 2000). In performance-avoidance, individuals construe the achievement setting as a threat and may try to escape the situation if the option is readily available. The prospect of potential failure elicits anxiety, encourages self-protective withdrawal of affective and cognitive resources, and orients the individual towards the presence of failure-relevant information processes hypothesized to undermine intrinsic motivation (Elliot & Harackiewicz, 1996).

Classroom Implications

A considerable body of evidence suggests motivation and learning are facilitated in settings that place a stronger emphasis on mastery rather than performance goals (Ames, 1992; Blumenfeld, 1992; Meece et al., 1988). The features of classes that induce either mastery or performance goal orientations include the following: the types of academic tasks that students are assigned, the type of classroom authority relationships, and the criteria used for evaluation and recognition (Ames, 1992).

Ames (1992) identified the classroom parameters that are associated with fostering mastery goals and those associated with fostering performance goals. Ames (1992) then argued that a classroom climate conductive to mastery goals is one in which both the student and teacher define success in terms of progress and improvement, place a high value on effort and learning, and view mistakes as part of the learning process. Other conditions that support mastery goals include: challenging tasks, a high degree of student choice and control, a focus on individual improvement and individual evaluation, and opportunities for students to work together on assignments (Ames, 1992; Maehr & Midgley, 1991). Classes with these characteristics engender greater student engagement in the learning processes and, therefore, higher levels of performance than do authoritarian classes that emphasize student ability comparisons and discourage collaboration (Karabenick & Collins-Eaglin, 1997). Conversely, a performance-oriented classroom is one in which success is defined by high grades, value is placed on high ability, and mistakes invoke anxiety in students (Ames, 1992; Anderman et al., 2002) In performance-oriented classrooms both students and the teacher are focused on the performance of the student relative to others (Ames & Archer, 1988).

Eppler and Harju (1997) noted that there needs to be a balance between mastery and performance goals both in terms of students' personal beliefs and the educational objectives that teachers develop and pursue. While mastery goals motivate students to engage in effective persistence, performance goals help students to set realistic expectations. Performance goals become problematic when there is too much focus on demonstrating one's ability rather than improving one's ability (Dweck, 1986).

Key to students' endorsement of achievement goals is how students interpret failure (Dweck, 1986; Eppler & Harju, 1997). From the mastery goal perspective, mistakes are a signal to try harder or to alter one's strategy. From the performance goal perspective, mistakes are a signal that one lacks ability and may as well give up trying. When students encounter difficult material or when they receive a poor score on an exam, there is a tendency to experience feelings of learned helplessness. These students may shy from academic challenges because they believe that making mistakes or exerting too much effort reflect low ability.

According to Eppler and Harju (1997) once instructors form an understanding of the impact of achievement goals on academic performance they might be able to help students identify their own beliefs about academic achievement and then encourage them to think about how these beliefs relate to performance. Furthermore, instructors may then be able to encourage students to increase their efforts and, even more important, explore alternative problem-solving strategies when they encounter academic obstacles (Eppler & Harju, 1997). Because achievement goals develop and change as students progress through the educational system, before educators can help students explore their motivational beliefs and how those beliefs impact educational outcomes, educators must first form a firm understanding of goal orientation from a developmental perspective.

A Developmental Perspective

There are a number of important reasons for examining goal orientation from a developmental perspective. First, there is a strong body of evidence indicating that acheivement motivation develops and changes over time (Anderman et al., 2002). For example, the intrinsic curiosity that young children have about the world around them often leads to interest in specific types of activities during childhood and adolescence thereby influencing motivation (Anderman et al., 2002). In addition, there is growing concern with grades and performance as students move through the educational system (Eccles, Wigfield, Harold, & Blumenfeld, 1993). Further, children, adolescents, and adults move through different educational contexts at different times. These contexts exert powerful effects on student motivation (Anderman et al., 2002).

There has been very little research on achievement goal orientation in young children. However, studies by Stipek and her colleagues (Stipek, Recchia, & McClintic, 1992) demonstrated that pre-school aged children experience feelings of shame in the face of failure. Cain and Dweck (1995) examined the motivational patterns of children in the first, third, and fifth grade. These researchers concluded that children in all three-grade levels showed concern about their ability and, therefore, could be classified as "helpless," thus having a performance orientation.

Nicholls (1979) demonstrated that children's conception of ability changes throughout childhood. While young children equate effort with ability, at about age 11 or 12, children are able to differentiate among concepts such as effort, ability, and performance. Dweck (1986) argued that when children are young and equate effort with ability, they might be more likely to be mastery oriented. Conversely, as children approach early adolescence and develop understandings of ability, effort, and performance, they may be more likely to adopt performance goals (Anderman et al., 2002).

During the adolescent years the endorsement of performance and mastery goals becomes particularly important because it leads to different outcomes. According to Anderman et al. (2002), these outcomes include the use of differing cognitive processing strategies, differing effects on learning, and differing approaches to academic tasks. These researchers also contended that the endorsement of mastery goals and performance goals by students change during the adolescent years. Students tend to endorse performance goals more often and mastery goals less as they progress through adolescence. This is particularly evident as students transition from elementary school to middle school, and research indicates that these shifts are due to changes in school goals (Anderman et al., 2002; Stipek, 2002). In a longitudinal study, Anderman and Anderman (1999) found that changes in individual achievement goals across middle school transitions were also related to perceptions of classroom goal structure.

As students progress through the educational system, the system tends to demand more of them (Anderman et al., 2002; Stipek, 2002). Whereas pre-school programs and elementary schools often do not focus on children's ability in comparison to the ability of others, as students progress through elementary school to secondary school, there is an increasing emphasis on ability, performance, and grades (Anderman et al., 2002; Stipek, 2002). This performance-oriented environment extends from high school into the college setting, where students compete for scholarships, graduate programs and eventually jobs. Although not all students progress to college, those who do may have learned to adapt to the increasingly performance-oriented demands of their educational environment (Anderman et al., 2002).

Collegiate populations, however, have not been studied extensively and it was not until the early 1990s that studies began to address achievement goals at the collegiate level (Harackiewicz et al., 1998, 2000; Hayamizu & Weiner, 1991; Miller et al., 1993; Roedal & Schraw, 1995; Schraw et al., 1995; Shields, 1993). Collegiate student populations are unique to study because there are important differences in the motivational attitudes of older and younger students that may impact their achievement goal orientation (Werring, 1987; Wolfgang & Dowling, 1981).

Shields (1993), for example, found that older students, at various stages in adult development, differed in their motivation for attending college and the personal satisfaction gained from the experience than their younger colleagues. Simply stated, Shields (1993) found that older students valued learning and wanted a college degree. While older students are more intrinsically motivated to acquire knowledge and develop competence in skills, younger students are more externally oriented toward forming social relationships, receiving external rewards, and living up to the expectations of others (Shields, 1993).

Differences in goal orientation in older and younger students may be tied to differences in ego and moral development (Burley et al., 1999). Loevinger (as cited by Burley et al., 1999) suggested that "as ego development proceeds through adulthood, individuals move away from externally derived standards and goals to internally derived standards and goals" (p. 85). Kohlberg (1976) argued that as individuals develop morally, they transition away from the desire to conform to the desires of peers and toward more individually determined ideas of right and wrong. These tendencies to move toward personally as well as internally derived standards with increasing age, according to Burley et al. (1999), may support the development of a mastery orientation in older students. Hence, individuals with more advanced ego development may pursue learning experiences for personal gratification rather than to satisfy the expectations of others (Burley et al., 1999).

Remarkably few studies exist that investigate the relationship of achievement goal orientation and student age at the collegiate level. One cross-sectional study that investigated only student age and achievement goal orientation, utilizing the *Goals Inventory*, suggested that significant differences exist in the adoption of goal orientation by older and younger students (Burley et al., 1999). Studying a sample of college students of diverse ages (17 through 59), Burley et al. (1999) concluded that the older students (25 years of age and older) were more mastery oriented than were the younger students. However, these researchers also recommended additional research.

Also utilizing the *Goals Inventory*, Eppler and Harju (1997) extended Dweck's (1986) model of achievement motivation to the collegiate level by examining the relationship between achievement goal orientation and academic performance. Unlike Burley et al. (1999), these researchers utilized the categories of "traditional" and "nontraditional" rather than "younger" and "older." The "traditional" and "nontraditional" categories, however, emphasized students' previous academic and work experience rather than student age. Moreover, the nontraditional category included participants ages 22 to 53. Although these researchers concluded that goal orientation was a better predicator of academic success than student status (traditional and nontraditional) and that nontraditional students endorsed mastery goals more strongly than their traditional peers, it was difficult to extrapolate the authors' interpretation of the data based on age.

In summary, studies that have investigated academic performance and achievement goal orientation in collegiate populations concluded that both mastery goals and performance goals may be beneficial (Eppler & Harju, 1997; Harakiewicz et al., 1997; Roedel & Schraw, 1995; Schraw et al., 1995). Specifically, these researchers found that students who endorsed mastery goals were more likely to indicate high levels of interest in the course materials at the end of the semester. The endorsement of performance goals predicted higher course grades. However, none of these researchers included student age in their studies. Therefore, the literature that addresses the relationship between achievement goal orientation and student age at the college level is limited to the study conducted by Burley et al. (1999). Thus, further research is warranted.

Summary

As demonstrated in the foregoing literature review, Dweck (1986) and Nicholl's (1984) models of achievement goal orientation laid the foundation for much of the research that has been conducted over the last 15-20 years in the realm of achievement motivation (Harackiewicz et al., 1998; Pintrich, 2000). These models are useful for understanding how attitudes relate to behavior in achievement situations. The above review has offered a historical review of the experimental and quasi-experimental literature that lead to the development and refinement of achievement goal theory.

Also examined was the current debate in the literature regarding which types of achievement goals promote optimal motivation. While a number of theorists endorsed a mastery goal perspective, focusing on the adaptive consequences of mastery goals and the maladaptive consequences of performance goals (Ames, 1992; Meece et al., 1988), others endorsed a multiple goal perspective in which both mastery and performance goals can be beneficial (Barron & Harackiewicz, 2001; Covington, 2000; Harackiewicz et al., 1998). Finally, the literature review addressed the impact of achievement goals in the classroom and offered a developmental perspective of achievement goals, thereby disclosing a gap in the literature concerning student age and achievement goal orientation at the collegiate level. This study addressed this gap in the literature by examining the relationship between achievement goal orientation and student age in physician assistant students.

Chapter 3 outlines the methodology and describes the study sample, variables, and instrumentation used in this study. Also discussed are the procedures for data collection and data analysis. Chapter 4 presents the findings of the study relative to the research questions. Finally, chapter 5 presents a summary of the study, as well as conclusions and recommendations for future research.

CHAPTER 3

METHODOLOGY AND RESEARCH DESIGN

Introduction

The purpose of this chapter is to describe the research design that guided this study. The design defined the framework for the research and delineated the types of statistical analyses that were conducted. Also included in this chapter is a discussion of the research questions and hypotheses and a description of the population and sample, instrumentation, and procedures selected for data collection and data analyses.

Research Design

The study employed a nonexperimental, quantitative design. According to Leedy and Ormrod (2001), "Quantitative research is used to answer questions about relationships among measured variables with the purpose of explaining, predicting, and controlling phenomenon" (p. 101). Given the nature of the problem and the need to explore the relationship between the variables of achievement motivation and student age, a correlational methodology was employed to answer the research questions.

For the purpose of data collection, the *Goals Inventory*, a Likert scale survey instrument, was utilized to assess the achievement goal orientation of the students. Often, Likert-type surveys are used to assess characteristics of a population and to determine the strength of the relationships among characteristics (Depoy & Gitlin, 1998; Likert, 1932). This data collection tool was judged advantageous by the investigator because it provides separate scores for mastery and performance goals. Also, the *Goals Inventory* specifically tests for mastery and performance goals rather than a combination of mastery/performance goals and approach/avoidance goals. The *Goals Inventory* is a validated instrument. Further validity and reliability data is offered in the Instrumentation section (Roedel et al., 1994)

The Spearman test and ANOVA were used to describe the nature of the relationship between achievement goal orientation and student age. Also, chi-square analysis was used to examine the differences in the goals students endorsed across the age cohorts. The chi-square test is a nonparametric procedure that compares the actual observed frequencies of a phenomenon within the sample with the frequencies that would be expected if there were no relationship between two or more variables in the population (Heiman, 1996).

Research Questions and Statistical Hypotheses

Research Question 1

What is the nature of the relationship between achievement goal orientation and student age?

H_O: There will exist no statistically significant relationship between mastery goals and student age.

H_A: There will exist a positive relationship between mastery goals and student age.

H_O: There will exist no statistically significant relationship between performance goals and student age.

H_A: There will exist a negative relationship between performance goals and student age.

Research Question 2

What is the difference in the achievement goals that students endorse across the age cohorts?

H_O: There will be no differences in the achievement goals that students endorse across the age cohorts.

H_A: Students in the "younger cohort" will endorse a high performance/low mastery goal orientation while students in the "middle cohort" and "older cohort" will endorse either a high mastery/low performance goal orientation or a high mastery/high performance goal orientation.

Population

The population for the study encompassed physician assistant students enrolled in accredited physician assistant programs nationwide as reported in the current list of accredited programs provided by the National Commission on Certification of Physician Assistants (Association of Physician Assistant Programs, 2001). The American Academy of Physician Assistants (1998) defines a physician assistant as a health care professional licensed to practice medicine with physician supervision. As part of their comprehensive responsibilities, "PAs conduct physical exams, diagnose and treat illnesses, order and interpret tests, counsel on preventive health care, assist in surgery, and, in most states, can write prescriptions" (American Academy of Physician Assistants, 1998, What is a PA? General Information Section).

Nationwide there are 143 accredited PA programs grouped in the following six consortia regions as defined by the American Association of Physician Assistant Programs: Northeastern, Eastern, Southeastern, Midwestern, Heartland, and Western

(Association of Physician Assistant Programs, 2002). These programs award either associate degrees, bachelor's degrees, master's degrees, and/or certificates of completion (Simon et al., 2002). Fifty-two of these programs offer a baccalaureate degree option.

Sample

For the purpose of this study, all 52 baccalaureate programs were invited to participate. Only baccalaureate programs were included for sampling because master's and certificate programs accept only students who already hold an undergraduate degree. Therefore, these programs, based on the experience of the researcher, attract an older student population than do baccalaureate programs. Further, only first-year PA students were included in the study. Thus, the researcher chose to limit the participant pool as a condition of control.

According to Simon et al. (2002), enrollment in first year PA classes averages 39 students per program nationwide (p. 38). Based on the above participant criteria, it was estimated that the projected sample pool would involve approximately 2,100 students. It was estimated that 50 % of the programs would agree to participate. Additionally, it was expected that 50 % of students in participating programs would participate. According to Babbie (1998) and Suskie (1996), a response rate of 50 % is adequate for analysis and reporting. Therefore, the expected sample size for the study was $N = 525$. However, of the 52 programs invited to participate, 20 programs completed the study. Therefore, the sample consisted of 499 students.

Variables

The first variable that was examined in the research procedure was achievement goal orientation. Achievement goal orientation represents an integrated pattern of beliefs that lead to different ways of approaching, engaging in, and responding to achievement situations (Ames, 1992). While mastery goals favor deep-level, strategic processing of information that lead to increased school achievement, performance goals trigger superficial, rote-level processing that exerts a stultifying influence on achievement (Dweck, 1986; Nicholls, 1984). Achievement goal orientation in this study was determined by the scores students achieved on the *Goals Inventory* (Appendix A).

The second variable that was examined is student age. For the purpose of data collection, students were asked to self-report their age on the Scantron form that the *Goals Inventory* was printed on. For the purpose of this study, the participant age data were disaggregated and grouped into three categories based on the trends in student demographics and attrition rates as reported by Simon et al. (2002). Participants who were less than 24 years of age were grouped into the "younger cohort" category while participants who were between the ages of 24 to 29 were grouped into a "middle cohort" category. Finally, participants older than 29 years of age were grouped into the "older cohort" category.

Instrumentation

The study utilized two data sources: The *Goals Inventory* and students' self-reported age.

Goals Inventory

The *Goals Inventory* was used to measure achievement goal orientation (Roedel et al., 1994). The *Goals Inventory* consists of 25 statements regarding attitudes and behaviors that reflect either mastery or performance goals as described by Dweck and Leggett (1988). The instrument includes 12 mastery goals statements, five performance goal statements, and eight filler statements that are not scored. The researcher omitted filler item eight, "I am willing to cheat to get a good grade," to avoid suspicion on the part of the students regarding the purpose of this study. Students were asked to rate how strongly each statement applied to them using a Likert scale (1 = never true; 5 = always true).

This instrument was primarily chosen because it provides separate scores for mastery and performance goals. These two variables are sometimes treated as if they were opposite endpoints of a single continuous dimension (Eison, 1981) rather than two independent factors as conceptualized by Dweck and Leggett (1988). This was an important consideration given the hypothesis that students in the "middle cohort" and in the "older cohort" would endorse either a high mastery/low performance goal orientation or a high mastery/high performance goal orientation.

Roedel et al. (1994) modeled the *Goals Inventory* on Schraw and Roedel's (1993) 48-item measure of goal orientation. Twenty-three items from this longer instrument were dropped on the basis of low factor loadings and/or item-to-total correlation (Roedel et al., 1994). Roedel et al. (1994) investigated the psychometric properties of the *Goals Inventory* and reported test-retest reliability [N = 187] for the mastery and performance goal scales as r = .73 for mastery goals subscale and r = .76 for the performance goals subscale. Internal consistency estimates were assessed using Cronbach's alpha. These values were reported as .80 and .75 respectively (Roedel et al., 1994).

Convergent and divergent validity were evaluated by comparing the *Goals Inventory* to the following instruments: *Reactions to Test*, which measured four dimensions of test-related anxiety; the *Hope Scale*, which measured two dimensions of hope as it relates to goal attainment; and the *Attribution Inventory*, which measured endorsement of 12 different causes for academic success and failure (Roedel et al., 1994). Correlations between the *Goals Inventory* and *Reactions to Tests* subscales supported Dweck and Leggett's (1988) prediction that high performance scores are associated with tension, worry, and high test anxiety whereas high mastery scores were not related to high test anxiety (Roedel et al., 1994). Correlations between the *Goals Inventory* and the *Hope Scale* matched the prediction that the mastery factor would correlate positively with the *Hope Scale* while the performance factor would correlate negatively (Roedel et al., 1994). Finally, correlations between the *Goals Inventory* and the *Attribution Inventory* matched the prediction attributions for academic success and failure would correlate with the mastery and performance factors in a manner analogous to that identified in Ames and Archer (1988).

Procedures for Data Collection

A letter of introduction was sent to the directors of all 52 baccalaureate physician assistant programs via electronic mail inviting participation in the study (Appendix B). This e-mail letter introduced the researcher, described the purpose of the study, and the requirements of the programs and students who chose to participate. The program directors that chose to participate were asked to complete and return to the researcher, via e-mail, a Program Information Form (Appendix C) in which they designated a "site coordinator" to aid in coordinating the data collection. Program directors were also asked to estimate the number of possible participants. Site coordinators received a packet containing the following items:

1. Instructions for the site coordinator (Appendix D).

2. Invitation to Participate/Consent Statements (Appendix E).

3. Survey instruments printed on Scantron forms.

4. Self-addressed, postage-paid return envelope.

The site coordinators were asked to read the Invitation to Participate/Consent Statement to the participants during a designated class period. The students who were willing to participate were given a copy of the Invitation to Participate/Consent Statement and a copy of the *Goals Inventory*. The participants were instructed to answer the question, "How old are you?" printed at the top of the Scantron form. After completing the instrument, students were asked to place the completed instruments in the self-addressed return envelope.

Site coordinators were asked to not collect the completed surveys but to let students place them in the envelope themselves to ensure confidentiality. Site coordinators were given 8 weeks to administer the surveys and return the completed Scantron sheets to the researcher. Three reminders were sent to the site coordinators by e-mail at 2-week intervals verifying the deadline. Consent by the participants was tacit; therefore, in accordance with Institutional Review Board policies, signed consent statements were not required.

Data Analysis

Characteristics of Data

The data collected for the variable of student age was treated as ordinal as students were grouped into one of three cohorts: "younger cohort," "middle cohort," and "older cohort." Data gathered from the *Goals Inventory* were placed into four categories of goal orientation. These categories are as follows: (1) Category A: low on performance and high on mastery (high-mastery group); (2) Category B: low on mastery and high on performance (high-performance group); (3) Category C: low on mastery and low on performance (both-low group); (4) Category D: high on mastery and high on performance (both-high group). These data were treated as nominal data. According to Heiman (1996), "with a nominal scale, each score does not actually indicate an amount; rather, it is used simply for identification" (p. 37).

Statistical Measures

To test the first hypothesis, both parametric and nonparametric statistical procedures were used. The first technique used to describe the relationship between achievement motivation and student age was the Spearman test, a nonparametric statistical procedure. The Spearman correlation coefficient is employed when data are treated as ordinal or rank-scores (Heiman, 1996). Also, to further explore the data analysis of variance (ANOVA) was computed. According to Heiman (1996), ANOVA is used to determine whether significant differences exist in experiments containing two or more sample means.

Using a median split of the mastery and performance goal scores, as suggested by Eppler and Harju (1997), the participants were placed into high/low categories for mastery goals and high/low categories for performance goals. All scores above the median were categorized as high for mastery/performance goals and all scores equal to or below the median were categorized as low for mastery/performance goals. To test the second hypothesis, chi-square analysis was employed. According to Heiman (1996), this test is often called the "test of independence" (p. 462).

Chi-square allows the researcher to make decisions about whether there is a relationship between two or more variables; if the null hypothesis is rejected, it is concluded that there is a statistically significant relationship between the variables. In this study, a measure of the strength of a relationship was computed using a Cramer's V test.

Social Change

Given the increasing market demand for physician assistants nationwide (Hecker, 2001), it was anticipated that the findings of this research would be of importance to physician assistant educators as they respond to the changing demographic and attrition patterns in their enrolling students as noted by Simon et al. (2002). Vago (1999) stated that institutions of higher education have a responsibility to respond to social change by preparing students to fully meet the needs of society. Understanding the relationship between achievement goal orientation and students age in physician assistant students at the college level may impact future curricular development as educators tailor courses and curricula to foster an atmosphere that better facilitates motivation and learning in their student population. Furthermore, educators may also be able to identify students at risk for academic hardships and develop effective intervention strategies (Eppler & Harju, 1997). Combined, these efforts may positively impact student retention rates, thereby lowering attrition.

Summary

The study examined the relationship between achievement goal orientation and student age. Outlined in this chapter were the research design, statistical hypotheses, and a description of the study population and sample. Also discussed were the study variables, instrumentation, and procedures for data collection and analyses. In the following chapter the analyses and interpretation of the data are presented. Finally, the conclusions of the study and the recommendations for future research are offered in chapter 5.

CHAPTER 4

RESULTS

Introduction

The purpose of this study was to examine the relationship between achievement goal orientation and student age in physician assistant (PA) students. Two research questions were addressed in this study. First, what is the nature of the relationship between achievement motivation and student age? Second, what is the difference in the achievement goals that students endorse across the age cohorts?

This study employed a nonexperimental, quantitative design. The sample consisted of first-year physician assistant students that were enrolled in accredited, baccalaureate degree physician assistant programs in the United States. Two types of data were collected: students' self-reported age and their achievement goal orientation as measured by the *Goals Inventory,* a validated, Likert-scale survey instrument (Roedel et al., 1994). This instrument consists of 24 statements regarding attitudes and behaviors that reflect either a mastery goal orientation or a performance goal orientation. Each orientation represents a different way of thinking about competence and creates a framework for how individuals approach, experience, and react to achievement situations (Ames & Archer, 1988; Dweck & Leggett, 1988; Nicholls, 1984).

Exploring the variable of student age as it relates to achievement goals in PA students is of particular importance given the trends in student age and attrition demographics noted by Simon et al. (2002). In the *18th Annual Report on Physician Assistant Educational Programs in the United States, 2001-2002,* Simon et al. (2002) noted an increased enrollment of students less than 24 years of age and of students between the ages of 24 and 29. Also noted was a decrease in the enrollment of students older than 29 years of age. Further, Simon et al. (2002) documented higher attrition rates for students between the ages of 20 to 23.

This chapter reports the results of the data analyses performed to test the three research hypotheses and is divided into three sections. The first section describes the sample. The second section presents a description of the data collected using the *Goals Inventory*. The final section presents the results of the analyses of the data for the three research hypotheses. The chapter concludes with a summary of the findings.

Description of the Sample

There are 52 colleges and universities in the United States that offer an accredited baccalaureate degree in physician assistant studies. All 52 programs were invited to participate in this study via an e-mail letter sent to the program directors. Twenty-six program directors (50%) returned the Program Informational Form and identified a site coordinator for the study, thereby agreeing to participate. Each of the site coordinators was subsequently sent a packet that contained the *Goals Inventory* printed on a Scantron sheet, instructions for the site coordinator on the background of the study and administration of the survey, the Invitation to Participate/Consent Statements for the students, and a self-addressed, postage-paid return envelope.

Site coordinators were given 8 weeks to administer the surveys and return the completed Scantron sheets to the researcher. Three reminders were sent to the site coordinators by e-mail at 2-week intervals verifying the deadline. Consent by participants was tacit; therefore, in accordance with Institutional Review Board policies, signed consent statements were not required. Of the 26 programs that agreed to participate, 20 programs (77%) returned the completed surveys. The site coordinators of the six programs that did not participate were contacted by telephone. Four site coordinators stated that the program experienced a change in leadership and could not participate. Two site coordinators stated they could not meet the deadline set for completion of the surveys.

According to Simon et al. (2002), enrollment in the first year PA classes average 39 students per program nationwide (p. 38). However, in this study, the mean class size was 32. As reported by the program directors on the Program Informational Form, there were 661 possible participants. A total of 543 students participated (82%). Of the students who participated, 531 answered the self-reported age question, "How old are you?" 500 completed the questions on mastery goal orientation, and 499 completed the questions on performance goal orientation. Therefore, the sample size for the study was $\underline{N}$ = 499.

The age of the participants ranged from 18 to 60, with a mean age of 28 and a standard deviation of 7.06. The median age of the participants was 26. For the purpose of this study, the participant age data were disaggregated and grouped into three categories based on the trends in student demographics and attrition rates as reported by Simon et al. (2002). Participants who were less than 24 years of age were grouped into the "younger cohort" category while participants who were between the ages of 24 to 29 were grouped into a "middle cohort" category. Finally, participants older than 29 years of age were grouped into the "older cohort" category.

The frequency distribution for the three age cohorts was calculated and is presented in Table 1. The student age distribution of the participants closely matched that reported by Simon et al. (2002), who found that students less than 24 years of age made up 27% of the surveyed programs nationwide, while students between the ages of 24 and 29 made up 39.7%, and older than 29 years of age made up 32.8% (p. 45). Thus, in terms of student age, the study sample was representative of the population, as reported by Simon et al. (2002).

Table 1

Frequency Distribution for the Age Cohorts

Age Cohorts	Frequency	%
Younger	138	26
Middle	223	42
Older	170	32
Total	531	100

Description of the Data Gathered From the Instrument

Table 2 presents the mean, median, and standard deviation scores for the mastery and performance goals as measured by the *Goals Inventory*. For mastery goals, scores ranged from 2.45 to 5.00, with a possible range of 1.0 to 5.0. For performance goals, scores ranged from 1.0 to 4.67, with a possible range of 1.0 to 5.0.

Table 2

Mean, Median, and Standard Deviation for Mastery and Performance Goal Scores

Goal Category	Mean	Median	Standard Deviation
Mastery	4.32	4.36	.413
Performance	2.89	2.83	.723

Using a median split of the mastery and performance goal scores as suggested by Eppler and Harju (1997), the participants were placed into high/low categories for mastery goals and high/low categories for performance goals. All scores above the median were categorized as high for mastery/performance goals and all scores equal to or below the median were categorized as low for mastery/performance goals. For mastery goals, of the 500 participants, 266 (53%) were categorized as low (at or below the median) and 234 (47%) were categorized as high (above median). For performance goals, of the 499 participants, 257 (52%) were placed in the low category and 242 (49%) were placed in the high category.

Testing the Research Hypotheses

Research Hypotheses 1 and 2

Research hypotheses 1 and 2 were derived from the first research question which asked, what is the nature of the relationship between achievement goal orientation and student age? Research Hypothesis 1 posits a positive relationship between mastery goals and student age. Research Hypothesis 2 posits a negative relationship between performance goals and student age. To test these hypotheses, both parametric and nonparametric statistical procedures were utilized. The first technique used to describe the relationship between achievement goal orientation and student age was the Spearman test, a non-parametric statistical procedure. The Spearman rank-order correlation coefficient describes the linear relationship between two variables using ranked scores (Heiman, 1996).

The Spearman correlation coefficient was computed using the three age cohorts and the high/low mastery and high/low performance goal categories. As presented in Table 3, for mastery goals the Spearman correlation coefficient was $r = .043$ and for performance goals the Spearman correlation coefficient was $r = -.114$. As hypothesized, these results indicated that a negative relationship existed between performance goals and student age. Amongst this group of participants, younger students had higher performance goal scores than their older peers and older students had higher mastery goal scores than their younger peers. The relationship between mastery goals and student age, however, was not statistically significant.

Table 3

Results of Spearman Correlation Test for Age Categories and Mastery and Performance Goals

	Mastery Goals	Performance Goals
Spearman's rho	.043	-.114
Sig. (2-tailed)	.332	.011
N	500	499

A deeper exploration of the data was done through one-way analysis of variance (ANOVA). ANOVA is a parametric statistical procedure for determining whether significant differences exist in an experiment containing two or more sample means (Heiman, 1996). The F statistic compares all sample means in a factor (independent variable) to determine whether two or more sample means represent different populations. When F is not significant, it indicates that there are no significant differences between any of the sample means; however, when the F statistic is significant, it indicates that there is a significant difference between the sample means (Heiman, 1996).

ANOVA was computed with age as the independent variable and the high/low mastery goals and the high/low performance goals, tested separately, as the dependent variable. For this statistical test, age was treated as a continuous variable. Results of the ANOVA computation for mastery and performance goals are presented in Table 4. ANOVA demonstrated that there was a statistically significant difference in the mean age of students endorsing a high mastery goal orientation and a low mastery goal orientation. Also demonstrated was a statistically significant difference in the mean age of students endorsing a high performance goal orientation and a low performance goal orientation. Although the Spearman test was not statistically significant for mastery goals and age, ANOVA confirmed that a statistically significant relationship existed between both age and mastery goals and age and performance goals.

Table 4

Results of the ANOVA for Mastery and Performance Goals and Student Age

		SS	df	MS	F	Sig.
Mastery	Between Groups	255.88	1	255.88	5.09	.024
	Within Groups	24970.79	497	50.24		
	Total	25226.68	498			
Performance	Between Groups	631.95	1	631.95	12.77	.000
	Within Groups	24594.73	497	49.49		
	Total	25226.68	498			

Research Hypothesis 3

Research Hypothesis 3 stated that participants in the "younger cohort" will endorse a high performance/low mastery orientation while participants in the "middle cohort" and "older cohort" will endorse either a high mastery/low performance orientation or a high mastery/high performance orientation. To test this hypothesis, a multiple goal approach, in which students can endorse a combination of mastery and performance goals was utilized (Butler & Winne, 1995; Harackiewicz et al., 1998; Pintrich & Garcia, 1991). Data gathered from the *Goals Inventory* were placed into four categories of goal orientation, as suggested by Eppler and Harju (1997). These categories are as follows: Category A: low on performance and high on mastery (high-mastery group); Category B: low on mastery and high on performance (high-performance group); Category C: low on mastery and low on performance (both-low group); Category D: high on mastery and high on performance (both-high group). Presented in Table 5 is the frequency distribution for goal categories and age categories.

Table 5

Frequency Distribution for Goal Categories and Age Categories

	Age Categories			
Goal Categories	Younger	Middle	Older	Total
A	27	43	52	122
B	36	62	32	130
C	32	61	42	135
D	37	43	32	112
Total	132	209	158	499

As indicated in Table 5, participants in the "younger cohort" endorsed a high performance/low mastery goal orientation and a high mastery/high performance goal orientation. These two goal orientations are at opposite ends of the achievement motivation spectrum with high mastery/high performance goals being adaptive (leading to positive achievement outcomes) and high performance/low mastery goals being maladaptive (leading to negative achievement outcomes) (Eppler & Harju, 1997). These results were puzzling and inconsistent with those reported by Eppler and Harju (1997) who reported that younger students consistently endorsed the maladaptive orientations of high performance/low mastery and low mastery/low performance.

The results for the "middle cohort," were inconsistent with the third research hypothesis. Students in this category endorsed high performance/low mastery goals and low mastery/low performance goals almost equally as strong. These two goal orientations are considered maladaptive (Eppler & Harju, 1997). Finally, as hypothesized, older students endorsed a high mastery/low performance orientation, an adaptive orientation. This result supported previous research by Burley et al. (1999) and Eppler and Harju (1997) who reported that mastery orientation is related to increasing age.

To determine whether distribution of participants in the goal categories is independent of the age categories, chi-square analysis was performed. The chi-square test is a nonparametric statistical known as the "test of independence" (Heiman, 1996, p. 462). Presented in Table 6 are the results of the chi-square test that demonstrated that there was a statistically significant difference in the goals students endorse across the age cohorts. Moreover, this test also demonstrated that the goal orientation of students was dependent on their age.

According to Heiman (1996) a significant chi-square indicates that there is a relationship between the variables being tested; however, further analyses must be computed to describe the strength of this relationship. To describe the strength of the relationship between the variables of age category and goal category, a Cramer's V correlation coefficient was computed. The value of the Cramer's V correlation coefficient ranges between 0 and 1.0 (Heiman, 1996). The closer the value is to 1.0, the greater the strength of the relationship between the variables. The Cramer's V correlation coefficient was .115 (p = .04) confirming that a statistically significant relationship existed between the variables of age and goal categories.

Table 6

Chi-Square Test

	Value	df	Sig.
Chi – Square	13.184	6	.040
N	499		

Summary

Based on the responses of 499 students from 20 physician assistant programs, this study sought to answer two research questions: (1) What is the nature of the relationship between achievement motivation and student age; (2) What are the differences in the goals that students endorse across the age cohorts? With respect to question number 1, the results of the data analyses demonstrated a positive relationship between age and mastery goals and a negative relationship between age and performance. Amongst the participants of this study, the older students had higher mastery goal scores than their younger peers, while younger students had higher performance goal scores than their older peers. Further, ANOVA demonstrated that there were significant differences in the mean age of students endorsing high/low mastery goals and high/low performance goals.

For Question 2, the analyses of the data for this sample indicated that across the three age cohorts the participants endorsed varying goals. While participants in the "older cohort" strongly endorsed high mastery/low performance goals, the participants in the "middle cohort" endorsed a high performance/low mastery goal orientation and a low mastery/ low performance goal orientation. Finally, results for the participants in the "younger cohort" were not as well defined as their peers. These participants endorsed a high performance/low mastery goal orientation as well as high mastery/high performance goal orientation equally as strong.

In chapter 5, the results of this study will be discussed and conclusions will be offered. Further, implications for social change will be explored. Finally recommendations for further research will be made.

CHAPTER 5

SUMMARY, CONCLUSIONS, AND RECOMMENDATIONS

Summary of Research Findings

Terrel Bell, former United States Secretary of Education, noted: "There are three things to remember about education. The first is motivation. The second one is motivation. The third one is motivation" (as quoted in Maehr & Meyer, 1997, p. 372). The concept of motivation stands at the center of the educational enterprise (Ames, 1992; Elliot & Harackiewicz, 1996). Contemporary research on achievement motivation is based largely on the analysis of the achievement goals that students adopt within the educational setting and the consequences of those goals on educational outcomes (Covington, 2000; Dweck, 1984; Harackiewicz, Barron, & Elliot, 1998; Nicholls 1984).

While numerous studies have investigated the relationship between achievement goal orientation and academic success at the collegiate level (Harackiewicz et al., 1998, 2000; Hayamizu & Weiner, 1991; Miller et al., 1993; Roedal & Schraw, 1995; Schraw et al., 1995; Shields, 1993), the review of the literature for this research identified only one study (Burley et al., 1999) that specifically addressed achievement motivation and student age. In an attempt to contribute to this limited body of literature, this study investigated the relationship between achievement goal orientation and student age in first year physician assistant (PA) students enrolled in accredited baccalaureate degree physician assistant programs in the United States.

This study employed a quantitative, nonexperimental design. The sample consisted of 499 participants from 20 PA programs. Two types of data were collected:

participants' self-reported age and their achievement goal orientation as measured by the *Goals Inventory*, a validated, Likert-scale survey instrument (Roedel et al., 1994).

Three research hypotheses were addressed in this study. Research Hypotheses 1 and 2 were derived from the first research question. Research Hypothesis 1 posited a positive relationship between mastery goals and student age. Research Hypothesis 2 posited a negative relationship between performance goals and student age. Results of the data analyses indicated that Research Hypotheses 1 and 2 were supported. While data analyses demonstrated a statistically significant relationship between performance goals and student age, the relationship between mastery goals and student age was not statistically significant, although it was in the expected direction in that older students had higher mastery goals scores than their younger peers. Further exploration of the data via ANOVA demonstrated that there existed a statistically significant difference in the mean age of students endorsing a high mastery goal orientation and a low mastery goal orientation. Also demonstrated was a statistically significant difference in the mean age of students endorsing a high performance goal orientation and a low performance goal orientation.

Research Hypothesis 3 stated that participants in the "younger cohort" would endorse a high performance/low mastery orientation while participants in the "middle cohort" and "older cohort" will endorse either a high mastery/low performance orientation or a high mastery/high performance orientation. Results of the data analyses provided partial support for Research Hypothesis 3. As hypothesized, participants in the "older cohort" endorsed a high mastery/low performance goal orientation. This goal orientation, according to Eppler and Harju (1997), is adaptive, leading to positive educational outcomes. Inconsistent with the hypothesized relationship, the participants in the "middle cohort" endorsed a high performance/low mastery goal orientation and a low performance/low mastery goal orientation. Both of these goal orientations are considered maladaptive, leading to negative educational outcomes (Eppler & Harju, 1997).

Results for participants in the "younger cohort" were also inconsistent with the third research hypothesis. Participants in this cohort endorsed both high mastery/high performance goals as well as high performance/low mastery goals. These goals, as reported by Eppler and Harju (1997), are at opposite ends of the achievement motivation spectrum with high mastery/high performance goals leading to positive educational outcomes and high performance/low mastery goals leading to negative educational outcomes.

In light of the foregoing summary of the results of the data analyses, this chapter begins by discussing these results in comparison to previous studies and draws several conclusions. Next, implications for social change are suggested. Finally, based on the results of this study, recommendations for further research are offered.

Conclusions from the Hypotheses

Research Hypotheses 1 and 2

Research Hypotheses 1 and 2 were derived from the first research question. The first research hypothesis posited a positive relationship between mastery goals and student age. The second research hypothesis posited a negative relationship between performance goals and student age. Results of the Spearman test for mastery and performance goals indicated that a positive relationship existed between mastery goals and student age and a negative relationship existed between performance goals and student age. Amongst this group of participants, younger students had higher performance goal scores than their older peers and older students had higher mastery goal scores than their younger peers. While the relationship for performance goals and age was statistically significant, the relationship between mastery goals and age was not.

Further exploration of the data was done through ANOVA. For both mastery goals and performance goals the results were significant. Results of the data analyses revealed significant differences in the mean ages of students in the high/low mastery goal categories as well as for those students in the high/low performance goal categories. While the results of the ANOVA corroborated those of Burley et al. (1999) as well as Eppler and Harju (1997), results of the Spearmen test did not fully support the findings of Burley et al. (1999). In contrast to the results of this study, Burley et al. (1999) reported a statistically significant correlation between age and mastery goals, while a weaker relationship was reported between age and performance goals.

One possible reason for the results obtained in this study, when compared to Burley et al. (1999), may be the way in which the age categories were conceptualized. While the participant age data for this study were grouped into three age categories based on the trends in student demographics and attrition rates as reported by Simon et al. (2002), Burley et al. (1999) and Eppler and Harju (1997) delineated only two age categories: older/younger and traditional/nontraditional. Although these categories are frequently discussed in the literature, as compared to the age categories used in this study, to adequately investigate the trends in PA education, as reported by Simon et al. (2002), this investigator chose to utilize three age cohorts. However, given the possibility that delineation of the age categories in this study may have influenced the results of the data analyses, an attempt was made to further explore the data from this study by regrouping the age data in a manner similar to that of previous researchers (Burley et al., 1999; Eppler & Harju, 1997).

Data for the "younger cohort" and for the "middle cohort" were collapsed into a single "younger cohort" category while the data for the "older cohort" remained unchanged. Although Burley et al. (1999) defined the "younger cohort" as students between the ages of 17 to 24 and the "older cohort" as students between the ages of 25 to 59, for the purposes of this analyses the "younger cohort" was defined as participants 29 years of age or younger and the "older cohort" as participants older than age 29. These categories were formed to more closely reflect the age groups discussed in Simon et al. (2002).

Using these revised age categories, the Spearman test was conducted. For mastery, $r = .086$ ($p = .056$). For performance, $r = -.109$ ($p = .015$). Again, the relationship between age and performance goals was significant, while the relationship between age and mastery goals was not. For mastery goals and age, however, there was a significant shift in the p-value from .332 to .056. Although a p-value of $> .05$ is not considered statistically significant (Heiman, 1996), the change in the p-value was remarkable. These results indicated that manipulation of the age categories might have significant implications for data analyses and thus interpretation of the results.

The differing results of the Spearman test for mastery goals and age obtained in this study, when compared to Burley et al. (1999), may also be due to a limitation of the Spearman test itself. The Spearman test is a nonparametric test that is not as sensitive as other tests (Heiman, 1996). However, the Spearman test is the only correlational test available for data that are categorical.

Research Hypothesis 3

Research Hypothesis 3 stated that participants in the "younger cohort" would endorse a high performance/low mastery orientation while participants in the "middle cohort" and "older cohort" would endorse either a high mastery/low performance orientation or a high mastery/high performance orientation. Results of the frequency distribution and chi-square analysis showed a statistically significant difference in the goals that students' endorsed across the age cohorts. Using a multiple goal approach in which participants can endorse a combination of mastery and performance goals, the findings of this additional analysis are presented by age categories below.

Younger Cohort and Middle Cohort

Students in the "younger cohort" endorsed a high performance/low mastery goal orientation almost as strongly as a high mastery/high performance goal orientation. These two goal orientations are at opposite ends of the achievement motivation spectrum with high mastery/high performance goals being adaptive, leading to positive achievement outcomes, and high performance/low mastery goals being maladaptive, leading to negative achievement outcomes (Eppler & Harju, 1997). These results were puzzling and inconsistent with those reported by Burley et al. (1999) and Eppler and Harju (1997). Burley et al. (1999) reported that younger students endorsed a performance goal orientation while their older peers endorsed a mastery goal orientation. Eppler and Harju (1997) reported that younger students more strongly endorsed a high performance/low mastery orientation or a low mastery/low performance orientation more than their older peers.

The results for the "middle cohort," although not as hypothesized, were less concerning and more consistent than the results for the "younger cohort." Participants in the "middle cohort" endorsed a high performance/low mastery goal orientation and a low mastery/low performance goal orientation almost equally as strong. These two goal orientations are considered maladaptive (Eppler & Harju, 1997). It is difficult to compare the findings of this cohort to either Burley et al. (1999) or Eppler and Harju (1997). Neither of these researchers delineated a "middle cohort"; rather, this cohort was considered part of the "younger cohort."

Of interest for both the "younger cohort" and "middle cohort" was the significant number of students who endorsed a low mastery/low performance goal orientation. As in Eppler and Harju's (1997) study, these students comprised a significant number of the sample size: 27 % of the entire sample. Although little is known about students who endorse this orientation, Eppler and Harju (1997) noted that students who rated both mastery and performance goals relatively low were least successful of all students and even less successful than those students who strongly endorsed performance goals. According to Eppler and Harju (1997), this group may be at a disadvantage academically because their efforts are guided by neither a desire for mastery nor anxiety about performance evaluation. Further, what motivates the students who endorse this orientation is unclear, but may need further explanation because, as Eppler and Harju (1997) noted, these students may be at risk for dropping out of college.

Older Cohort

Results of the data analyses for students in the "older cohort" were as hypothesized. Students in this age cohort strongly endorsed a high mastery/low performance orientation, an adaptive orientation. This result corroborates previous research by Burley et al. (1999), who reported that mastery orientation is related to increasing age. According to Burley et al. (1999), as students age they become more aware of the importance of knowledge and mastery of a topic and less concerned about external evaluation. Further, because ego development may influence the decision of an individual to pursue learning, individuals with more advanced ego development may pursue education for personal reasons rather than to fulfill the expectations that others may hold for them (Burley et al., 1999).

The fact that older students strongly endorsed mastery goals is also consistent with Shields (1993), who reported that older students place a high value on learning and mastery of knowledge and skills for its own sake. These findings also support the reports by Werring (1987) and Wolfgang and Dowling (1981) that older students have a higher level of intrinsic motivation than younger students who are more concerned with external evaluations and living up to the expectations of others.

Revised Age Categories

As in Research Hypotheses 1 and 2, the possibility that the delineations of the age cohorts affected the results of the data analyses was considered. Table 7 presents the frequency distribution for these revised age categories. For this new grouping, chi-square analysis was conducted. The chi-square value was 10.27 ($p = .016$). Again, results of the chi-square demonstrated a statistically significant difference in the goals that students endorse across the age cohorts. To describe the strength of the relationship between age category and goal category, a Cramer's V correlation coefficient was computed. The Cramer's V correlation coefficient was .143 (p =.016). The Cramer's V confirmed that a statistically significant relationship existed between the variables of age and goal categories.

Table 7

Revised Frequency Distribution for Age Categories and Goal Categories

Goal Category	Younger	Older	Total
A	70	52	122
B	98	32	130
C	93	42	135
D	80	32	112
Total	341	158	499

As displayed in Table 7, when the data for the "younger" and "middle" cohorts were collapsed, students in this revised "younger cohort" strongly endorsed either a high performance/low mastery goal orientation or a low mastery/low performance goal orientation. These two goal orientations, according to Eppler and Harju (1997), are maladaptive. For participants in the "older cohort" the results remained unchanged. These participants strongly endorsed a high mastery/low performance orientation. This orientation, according to Eppler and Harju (1997), is considered adaptive.

The results of the data analyses for the revised age categories more closely reflect the results of the previous studies (Burley, 1999; Eppler & Harju, 1997). The differences seen in the goals that younger students endorse, when considered separately from the "middle cohort" and when combined with the "middle cohort," are significant in terms of data interpretation. From a theoretical perspective, while the findings observed by combining the younger and middle cohorts are more consistent with the literature and more closely match those reported by previous researchers (Burley et al., 1999; Eppler & Harju, 1997), results of data analyses employing three age cohorts (younger, middle, and older) are confusing for participants in the younger cohort.

Delineation of the Age Cohorts

As demonstrated above, there exists a relationship between student age and achievement goal orientation. For mastery goals and student age, there was a positive relationship, while for performance goals and student age, there was a negative relationship. Also, it is evident that students endorsed different goals across the age cohorts. Intuitively, these finding are expected given that older students, at various stages in adult development, differ in their motivation for attending college and the personal satisfaction gained from the experience than their younger colleagues (Shields, 1993). From a developmental perspective, however, the findings are also not surprising. There is a strong body of evidence indicating that academic motivation develops and changes over time as children, adolescents, and adults move through different educational contexts at different times (Anderman et al. 2002). These contexts exert powerful effects on student motivation.

As discussed in the conclusions section of this chapter, the delineation of the age cohorts played an important role in the data analyses and interpretation. In the process of formulating the research design and the variables that were examined in this study, this researcher conducted an extensive search of the educational, psychological, and sociological literature utilizing a number of databases. To search the psychological literature the following databases were utilized: PsychInfo and PsychArticles. To search the sociological literature, Sociological Abstracts was utilized. To search the educational literature, ERIC and Educational Abstracts were utilized. Finally, to search the medical literature, Medline and CINAHL were used. The following keywords guided the search: motivation, achievement motivation, achievement goals, need achievement theory, intrinsic motivation, academic performance, higher education, student age, adult development, developmental stages, age differences, adult education, and psychosocial development.

Throughout the educational, psychological, and sociological literature, two sets of age categories have been studied in adult education: older students/younger students and traditional students/nontraditional students. These categories mirror the age categories studied by Burley et al. (1999) and Eppler and Harju (1997). No additional studies could be identified in the literature that went beyond these categories and examined adult learners utilizing the three age categories examined in this study. Specifically, no studies were found that addressed the "middle cohort" as defined by Simon et al. (2002).

The three age cohorts utilized in this study were formed based on current trends in PA student demographics and attrition rates (Simon et al., 2002). According to Simon (personal communication, February 25, 2002), the age categories delineated in the *18th Annual Report on Physician Assistant Educational Programs in the United States, 2000-2001* were formed to better facilitate the surveillance of trends in PA education rather than for theoretical reasons. Although, the findings of this study corroborate the findings of Eppler and Harju (1997) and Burley et al. (1999) for older students, for this study the results were not as clear for students in the "younger" and "middle" cohorts. Lacking a rich literature base with which to compare the results of this study to, it was difficult to make further conclusions concerning the middle and younger cohorts. It is evident, however, that the delineation of the age cohorts may be an important consideration for future research.

Implications for Social Change

The results of this study, like those of Burley et al. (1999) and Eppler and Harju (1997), demonstrated that there exist differences in the goals that students endorse across the age cohorts. While older students endorse mastery goals more strongly than their younger peers, younger students endorse performance goals more strongly than their older peers. These findings are important for PA educators given the rapidly changing demographics of students enrolling in PA programs as reported by Simon et al. (2002) in the *18th Annual Report on Physician Assistant Educational Programs in the United States, 2001-2002*. Simon et al. (2002) reported an increased enrollment of younger students, while the enrollment of older students, those older than 29 years of age, has systematically decreased over the last four years. This report also documented higher attrition rates for students in the younger cohort in comparison to their older peers.

Vago (1999) stated that institutions of higher education have a responsibility to respond to social change by preparing students to fully meet the needs of society. Given the rising demand for qualified PAs to meet the needs of an aging public and an overwhelmed health care system (Berman, 2001; Hecker, 2001), PA educators must evaluate their courses and curricula and possibly restructure them to better reflect an atmosphere which fosters motivation and learning for their students.

Ames (1992) suggested that motivation and learning are facilitated by certain classroom characteristics such as the types of academic tasks students are assigned, classroom authority, and the criteria used for evaluation and recognition. Further, Ames (1992) reported that a classroom climate conductive to mastery goals is one in which both the student and teacher define success in terms of progress and improvement, place a high value on effort and learning, and view mistakes as part of the learning process. Other conditions that support mastery goals include challenging tasks, a high degree of student choice and control, a focus on individual improvement and individual evaluation, and opportunities for students to work together on assignments (Ames, 1992; Maehr & Midgley, 1991). Taking this into account, PA educators must now respond by developing strategies to improve student learning and to encourage the development of mastery goals.

One strategy instructors can use to encourage mastery goals in the younger student population is to encourage younger students to interact and work with their older peers (Burley et al., 1999). By working together, younger students may observe older students and model mastery-oriented behaviors, such as asking questions that go beyond the test material and pursuing information not required for the class (Burley, 1999; Eppler & Harju, 1997). According to Eppler and Harju (1997), educators can further encourage mastery goal orientation by structuring class time so that students are more actively involved in the learning process.

Assignments can also be developed where students must apply abstract ideas in real-life context. In PA education, problem-based learning and cooperative learning are ideal for encouraging students not only to work together, but also to consider the real-life application of the material being studied. Although these forms of teaching have become popular over the last 5 years, many educators are resistant to these new methodologies (Tennant & Pogson, 1995).

Successful restructuring of courses and curricula rely on a commitment not only from instructors, but also from administrators. Resistance to change by seasoned faculty must be met with an equal commitment to change by administrators. However, given the results of this study, the increasing market demand for physician assistants nationwide (Hecker, 2001), and the rapidly changing demographics of students enrolling in PA programs, educators may now be more willing to make curricular changes to better serve their student population if not with less resistance, possibly with an improved understanding of the impact of student age on achievement motivation, and, thus, on academic outcomes. Combined, these efforts may positively impact student retention rates, thereby lowering attrition.

Recommendations

The motivation of college-aged individuals has been virtually neglected in the achievement motivation literature (Burley et al., 1999; Eppler & Harju, 1997; Maehr & Meyer, 1997). In fact, it was not until the early 1990s that studies began to address achievement goals at the collegiate level (Harackiewicz et al., 1998, 2000; Hayamizu & Weiner, 1991; Miller et al., 1993; Roedal & Schraw, 1995; Schraw et al., 1995; Shields, 1993). As discussed earlier, the review of the literature identified only one study (Burley et al., 1999) that specifically addressed the topic of achievement motivation and student age at the collegiate level.

Collegiate populations differ from elementary and secondary school populations in that in collegiate populations there exists a heterogeneous population of older and younger students. Researchers contend that important differences exist in the motivational attitudes of older and younger students that may impact their achievement motivation and, hence, their academic performance (Burley et al., 1999; Werring, 1987; Wolfgang & Dowling, 1981). Given an aging population that continually needs to have its knowledge and skills updated, it is important to pay attention to the motivation and learning patterns of adults (Maehr & Meyer, 1997). Future research should utilize longitudinal research designs to track developmental changes in the motivational and learning patterns of students as they progress through college. According to Maehr and Meyer (1997), researchers know little about motivation as a life-long process and they need to consider how these concepts, that frame motivational life, develop throughout the lifespan.

Questions still remain on the best method to study student age. Specifically, delineating the age cohorts to be studied is challenging. Three age cohorts were utilized in this study: the "younger cohort" (students less than 24 years of age), the "middle cohort" (students 24 to 29 years of age), and the "older cohort" (students older than 29 years of age). Conversely, Burley et al. (1999) studied two age groups: the "younger" group (students between ages 17 to 24) and the "older" group (those between the ages 25 to 59). Finally, Eppler and Harju (1997) studied age as a variable within the "traditional" and "nontraditional" student status. Here students in the "traditional" status were less than 22 years of age and those in the "nontraditional" status were between 22 and 53 years of age. Thus, there is much variation in the definition of older and younger students throughout the literature.

Future research needs to focus on refining methodologies for studying student age and achievement motivation. Clearer definitions of "younger" and "older" students are needed. Future research should also investigate the existence of a "middle" cohort outside of PA education and how motivational patterns of students in this cohort differ from their peers. With clearer definitions of student age, further research is needed to answer the question, "What is the precise age at which mastery goals becomes more valued to a student than performance goals?"

Future research should also focus on students who endorse a low mastery/low performance goal orientation. According to Eppler and Harju (1997), little is know about students who endorse this goal orientation. As in Eppler and Harju's (1997) study, these students composed a significant number of the sample size: 27 % of the entire sample. According to Eppler and Harju (1997), this group may be at a disadvantage academically because their efforts are guided by neither a desire for mastery nor anxiety about performance evaluation. Further, what motivates the students who endorse this orientation is unclear, but may need further explanation because these students may be at risk for dropping out of college (Eppler & Harju, 1997).

Finally, although gender, socioeconomic status, culture, ethnicity, previous academic experience, and previous health care experience may impact motivation, this study did not investigate these variables. Further research studying the effects of these variables on achievement motivation, at the collegiate level, should also be conducted.

References

Ainley, M.D. (1993). Styles of engagement with learning: Multidimensional assessment of their relationship with strategy use and school achievement. *Journal of Educational Psychology, 85,* 395-405.

American Academy of Physician Assistants. (1998). *What is a PA? General Information.* Retrieved October 2, 2001 from http://www.aapa.org/geninfo1.html

Ames, C. (1984). Achievement attributions and self-instructions under competitive and individualistic goal structures. *Journal of Educational Psychology, 76,* 478-487.

Ames, C. (1992). Classrooms: Goals, structures, and student motivation. *Journal of Educational Psychology, 84,* 261-271.

Ames, C., & Ames, R. (1984). Systems of student and teacher motivation: Toward a qualitative definition. *Journal of Educational Psychology, 76,* 535-556.

Ames, C. & Archer, J. (1988). *Achievement goals in the classroom: Student learning strategies and motivation processes,* Paper presented at the annual meeting of the American Education Research Association. Washington DC.

Anderman, L.H. & Anderman, E.M. (1999). Social predicators of change in students' achievement goal orientations. *Contemporary Educational Psychology, 25,* 21-37.

Anderman, E. M., Austin, C.C., & Johnson, D.M. (2002). The development of goal orientation. In A. Wigfield & J.S. Eccles (Eds.), *Development of Achievement Motivation* (pp. 197-223). San Diego, CA: Academic Press.

Association of Physician Assistant Programs (2001). *2001 Physician assistant programs directory (19th ed.).* Alexandria, VA: APAP.

Association of Physician Assistant Programs (2002). *Physician Assistant Program Directory.* Retrieved October 1, 2002 from http://.apap.org/apapdirectory/login.asp

Atkinson, J.W. (1957) Motivational determinants of risk-taking behavior. *Psychology Review, 64,* 359-372.

Babbie, E. (1998). *The practice of social research (8th Ed).* Belmont, CA: Wadswoth Publishing Company.

Barron, K.E., & Harackiewicz, J.M. (2001). Achievement goals and optimal motivation: Testing multiple goal models. *Journal of Personality and Social Psychology, 80*(5), 706.

Berman, M.J. (2001). Industry output and employment projections to 2010. *Monthly Review, 124* (11), 39-56.

Blumenfeld, P.C. (1992). Classroom learning and motivation: clarifying and expanding goal theory. *Journal of Educational Psychology, 84*(3), 272-281.

Bouffard, T., Boisvert, J., Vezeau, C., & Larouche, C. (1995). The impact of goal orientation on self-regulation and performance among college students. *British Journal of Educational Psychology, 65,* 317-329.

Burley, R.C., Turner, L.A., & Vitulli, W.F. (1999). The relationship between goal orientation and age among adolescents and adults. *Journal of Genetic Psychology, 160*(1), 84-89.

Butler, R. (1987). Task-involving and ego-involving properties of evaluation: Effects of different feedback conditions on motivational perceptions, interest, and performance. *Journal of Educational Psychology, 79,* 474-482.

Butler, D., & Winne, P. (1995). Feedback and self-regulated learning: A theoretical synthesis. *Review Educational Research, 65,* 245-281.

Cain, K., & Dweck, C.S. (1995). The relationship between motivational patterns and achievement cognitions through the elementary school years. *Merrill-Palmer Quarterly, 41*(1)1995 p.25-52.

Covington, M.V. (2000). Goal theory, motivation, and school achievement: An integrative review. *Annual Review of Psychology, 51,* 171-200.

Deci, E.L., & Ryan, R.M. (1985). *Intrinsic motivation and self-determination in human behavior.* New York, NY: Plenum.

Depoy, E. & Gitlin, L.N. (1998). *Introduction to research: Understanding and applying multiple strategies.* St. Louis, MO: Mosby.

Dweck, C.S. (1986). Motivational processes affecting learning. *American Psychologist, 41,* 1040-1048.

Dweck, C.S., & Bempechat, J. (1983). Children's theories of intelligence: Consequences for learning. In S. Paris, G. Olsen, & S. Stevenson (Eds.), *Learning and motivation in the classroom* (pp. 239-256). Hillsdale, NJ: Erlbaum.

Dweck, C.S., & Elliot, E.S. (1983). Achievement motivation. In E.M. Hetherington (eds.), *Socialization, personality, and social development* (pp. 643-691). NY: Wiley.

Dweck, C.S. & Leggett, E.L. (1988). A social cognitive approach to motivation and personality. *Psychology Review, 95*, 256-273.

Eccles, J.S., Wigfield, A., Harold, R., & Blumenfeld, P. (1993). Age and gender differences in children's self and task perceptions during elementary school. *Child Development, 64*, 830-847.

Eison, J.A. (1981). A new instrument for assessing students' orientation towards grades and learning. *Psychological Reports, 48*, 919-924.

Elliot, A.J., & Church, M. (1997). A hierarchal model of approach and avoidance achievement motivation. *Journal of Personality and Social Psychology, 72*, 218-232.

Elliot, A.J., & Harackiewicz, J.M. (1996). Approach and avoidance intrinsic goals and achievement motivation: A mediational analysis. *Journal of Personality and Social Psychology, 70*, 968-980.

Eppler, M.A., & Harju, B.L. (1997). Achievement motivation goals in relation to academic performance in traditional and nontraditional college students. *Research in Higher Education, 38*(5), 557-573.

Graham, S., & Golan, S. (1991). Motivational influences on cognition: Task involvement, ego involvement, and depth of information processing. *Journal of Educational Psychology, 83*, 187-194.

Harackiewicz, J.M., Barron, K.E., & Elliot, A.J. (1998). Rethinking achievement goals: When are they adaptive to college students and why? *Educational Psychology, 33*, 1-21.

Harackiewicz, J.M., Barron, K.E., Carter, S.M., Lehto, A.T., & Elliot, A.T. (1997). Predicators and consequences of achievement goals in the college classroom: Maintaining interest and making the grade. *Journal of Personality and Social Psychology, 73* (6), 1284-1295.

Harackiewicz, J.M., Barron, K.E., Tauer, J.M., Carter, S.M., & Elliot, A.J. (2000). Short-term and long-term consequences of achievement goals: Predicting continued interest and performance overtime. *Journal of Educational Psychology, 92*, 315-330.

Harackiewicz, J.M., & Elliot, A.J. (1993). Achievement goals and intrinsic motivation. *Journal of Personality and Social Psychology, 65*(5), 904-915.

Hayamizu, T., & Weiner, B. (1991). A test of Dweck's model of achievement goals as related to perceptions of ability. *Journal of Experimental Education, 59*, 226-234.

Hecker, E.D. (2001). Occupational employment projections. *Monthly Labor*

Review, 124 (11), 57-84.

Heiman, G.W. (1996). *Basic statistics for the behavioral scientist.* Boston, MA: Houghton Mifflin Company.

Karabenick, S.A., & Collins-Eaglin, J. (1997). Relation of perceived instructional goals and incentives to college students use of learning strategies. *Journal of Experimental Education, 65* (4), 331-341.

Koestner, R., Zuckerman, M., & Koestner, J. (1989). Attributional focus of praise and children's intrinsic motivation: The moderating role of gender. *Personality and Social Psychology Bulletin, Vol. 1, 15*(1), 61-72.

Kholberg, L. (1976). Moral stages and moralization: The cognitive-developmental approach. In J. Lickona (Ed.), *Moral development behavior: Theory, research, and social issues.* New York: Holt, Rinehart, Winston.

Leedy, P.D., & Ormrod, J.E. (2001). *Practical research: planning and design (7th ed.).* Upper Saddle River, NJ: Merrill Prentice Hall.

Lewin, K., Dembo, T., Festinger, L., & Sears, P.S. (1944). Levels of aspiration. In J. McHunt (Eds.), *Personality and the behavior disorders* (Vol. 1, pp. 333-378). NY: Ronald Press.

Likert, R. A. (1932). Technique for the Measurement of Attitudes. *Archives of Psychology*, 140.

Maehr, M.L. (1989). Thoughts about motivation. In C. Ames and R. Ames (Eds.), *Research on motivation in education: Goals and cognition* (Vol. 3, pp. 299-315). NY: Academic Press.

Maehr, M.L., & Meyer, H.A. (1997). Understanding motivation and schooling: Where we've been, where we are, and where we need to go. *Educational Psychology Review, 9*, 371-409.

Maehr, M.L., & Midgley, C. (1991). Enhancing school motivation: A school-wide approach. *Educational Psychologists, 26*, 399-427.

Maehr, M.L., & Nicholls, J.G. (1980). Culture and achievement motivation. In N. Warren (Ed.), *Studies in cross-cultural psychology* (Vol. 2, pp. 221-267). NY: Academic Press.

McClelland, D.C. (1951). Measuring motive in phantasy. In H. Guetzkow (Eds.), *Groups, leadership, and men* (pp. 191-205). Pittsburg, PA: Carnegie Press.

Meece, J.L., Blumenfeld, P.C., & Hoyle, R.H. (1988). Students' goals, orientations, and cognitive engagement in classroom activities. *Journal of Educational Psychology, 80,* 514-523.

Meece, J.L., & Holt, K. (1993). A pattern analysis of students' achievement goals. *Journal of Educational Psychology, 85,* 582-590.

Middleton, M.J., & Midgley, C. (1997). Avoiding the demonstration of lack of ability: An under explored aspect of goal theory. *Journal of Educational Psychology, 89,* 710-718.

Miller, R.B., Brehens, J.T., Greene, B.A., & Newman, D. (1993). Goals and perceived ability: Impact on student valuing, self-regulation, and persistence. *Contemporary Educational Psychology, 18,* 2-14.

Nicholls, J.G. (1979). Quality and inequality in intellectual development. *American Psychologist, 34,* 1071-1084.

Nicholls, J.G. (1984). Achievement motivation: Conceptions of ability, subjective experience, task choice, and performance. *Psychology Review, 91,* 328-346.

Nicholls, J.G., Patashick, M., Cheung, P., Thorkildsen, T.A., & Lauer, J.M. (1989). Can achievement motivation theory succeed with only one conception of success? In F. Halisch and J. Vanden Beroken (Eds.), *International perspective on achievement motivation* (pp. 187-208). Lisse, Netherlands: Swets and Zeitlinger.

Nolan, S.B. (1988). Reasons for studying: Motivational orientations and study strategies. *Cognition and Instruction, 5*(4), 269-287.

Pintrich, P.R. (2000). Multiple goals, multiple pathways: The role of goal orientation in learning and achievement. *Journal of Educational Psychology, 92*(3), 544-555.

Pintrich, P.R., & De Groot, E. (1990). Motivational and self-regulated learning components of classroom academic performance. *Journal of Educational Psychology, 82,* 33-40.

Pintrich, P.R., & Garcia, T. (1991). Student goal orientation and self-regulation in the college classroom. In M.J., Maehr & P.R. Pintrich (Eds.) *Advances in motivation and achievement: goals and self-regulatory process* (Vol. 7, pp. 371-402). Greenwich, Ct: JAI.

Pintrich, P.R., Roeser, R., & De Groot, E. (1994). Classroom and individual differences in early adolescents' motivation and self-regulated learning. *Journal of Early Adolescence, 14,* 139-161.

Pintrich, P.R., & Schrauben, B. (1992). Students' motivational beliefs and their cognitive engagement in classroom tasks. In D.H. Schunk & J. Meece (Eds.), *Student perception in the classroom: causes and consequences.* (pp. 149-183). Hillsdale, NJ: Lawerence Erlbaum Associates.

Pokay, P., & Blumenfeld, P.C. (1990). Predicting achievement early and late in the semester: the role of motivation and use of learning strategies. *Journal of Educational Psychology, 82*, 41-50.

Rawsthorne, L.J., & Elliot, A.J. (1999). Achievement goals and intrinsic motivation: meta-analytic review. *Personality and Social Psychology Bulletin, 3*(4), 326.

Roberts, G.C. (1992). *Motivation in sports and exercise* (pp. 3-29). Champaign, Il: Kinetics.

Roedel, T.D., & Schraw, G. (1995). Beliefs about intelligence and academic goals. *Contemporary Educational Psychology, 20*, 464-468.

Roedel, T.D., Schraw, G., & Plake, B.S. (1994). Validation of a measure of learning and performance goal orientations. *Educational and Psychological Measurement, 54*, 1013-1021.

Ryan, R.M. (1982). Control and information in the intrapersonal sphere: An extension of cognitive evaluation theory. *Journal of Personality and Social Psychology, 43*, 450-461.

Ryan, R. M. (1992). Agency and organization: Intrinsic motivation, autonomy, and the self in psychological development. In R. Dienstbier (Eds.), *Nebraska Symposium on Motivation* (Vol. 38, pp. 1-56). Lincoln, NK: University of Nebraska Press.

Ryan, R.M., Koestner, R., & Deci, E.L. (1991). Ego-involved persistence: When free-choice behavior is not intrinsically motivated. *Motivation and Emotion, 15*(3), 185-205.

Ryan, R.M. & Stiller, J. (1991). The social context of internalization: Parent and teacher influences on autonomy, motivation, and learning. In M.L. Maehr & P.R. Pintrich (Eds.), *Advances in motivation and achievement* (Vol. 7, pp. 115-149). Greenwich, CT: JAI.

Schraw, G., & Roedel, T.D.(1993, April).*Beliefs about intelligence and academic goals.* Poster presented at the meeting of the American Educational research Association, Atlanta, GA.

Schraw, G., Horn, C., Thorndike-Christ, T., & Bruning, R. (1995). Academic goal orientations and student classroom achievements. *Contemporary Educational Psychology, 20*, 359-368.

Shields, N. (1993). Attribution processes and stages of adult life development among adult university students. *Journal of Applied Social Psychology, 23,* 1321-1336.

Simon, A., Link, M., & Miko, A. (2002). *Eighteenth annual report on physician assistant educational programs in the United States, 2000-2001.* Alexandria, VA: Association of Physician Assistant Programs.

Skaalvik, E. (1997). Self-enhancing and self-defeating ego orientation: Relations with task and avoidance orientation, achievement, self-perceptions, and anxiety. *Journal of Educational Psychology, 89,* 71-81.

Stipek, D., Recchia, S., & McClintic, S. (1992). Self-evaluation in young children. *Monographs of Society for Research in Child Development, 57* (1, Serial No. 226).

Stipek, D. (2002). *Motivation to learn: Integrating theory and practice (4th Ed).* Boston: Allyn And Bacon.

Suskie, L.A. (1996). *Questionnaire survey research: What works (2nd Ed).* Tallahassee, Fl: Association for Institutional Research.

Tennant, M., & Pogson, P. (1995). *Learning and change in the adult years: A developmental perspective.* San Francisco: Jossey-Bass Publishers.

Vago, S. (1999). *Social change* (4th ed.) Upper Saddle River, New Jersey: Prentice Hall.

Vander Zanden, J.W. (1987). *Social psychology (4th Ed).* New York: Random House.

Wentzel, K.R. (1993). Motivation and achievement in early adolescence: The role of multiple classroom goals. *Journal of Early Adolescence, 13,* 4-20.

Werring, C.J. (1987). Responding to the older aged full-time student: Preferences for undergraduate education. *College Student Affairs Journal,* 13-20.

Wolfgang, M.E., & Dowling, W.D. (1981). Differences in motivation of adult and younger undergraduates. *Journal of Higher Education, 52,* 640-648.

Wolters, C.A. (1998). Self-regulated learning and college students' regulation of motivation. *Journal of Educational Psychology, 90(2),* 224-235.

Wolters, C.A., Yu, S.L., & Pintrich, P.R. (1996). The relationship between goal orientation and students' motivational beliefs and self-regulated learning. *Learning Individual Differences*, 8, 211-238.

Zimmerman, B.J. (1990). Self-regulated learning and academic achievement: An overview. *Educational Psychologists, 25*, 3-17.

Appendix A

Goals Inventory Questionnaire

ATTENTION STUDENTS: PLEASE DO NOT PUT YOUR NAME ON THIS SHEET.

HOW OLD ARE YOU? _____

Please answer the following questions by indicating how true each statement is about your experiences as a student on a scale of 1-5.

	Never True		Neutral		Always True
I enjoy challenging school assignments.	1	2	3	4	5
It is important for me to get better grades than my classmates.	1	2	3	4	5
I persevere even when I am frustrated by a task.	1	2	3	4	5
Academic success is largely due to effort.	1	2	3	4	5
Sticking with a challenging task is rewarding.	1	2	3	4	5
I try even harder after I fail at something.	1	2	3	4	5
I adapt well to challenging circumstances.	1	2	3	4	5
I work hard even when I don't like a class.	1	2	3	4	5
I am very determined to reach my goals.	1	2	3	4	5
Personal mastery of a subject is important to me.	1	2	3	4	5
I work very hard to improve myself.	1	2	3	4	5
I like others to think I know a lot.	1	2	3	4	5
It bothers me the whole day when I make a big mistake.	1	2	3	4	5
I feel angry when I do not do as well as others.	1	2	3	4	5
I am naturally motivated to learn.	1	2	3	4	5
I prefer challenging tasks even if I don't do as well at them.	1	2	3	4	5
Every student can learn to be a successful learner.	1	2	3	4	5
Learning can be judged best by the grade one gets.	1	2	3	4	5
My grades do not necessarily reflect how much I learn.	1	2	3	4	5
Mistakes are a healthy part of learning.	1	2	3	4	5
I feel most satisfied when I work hard to achieve something.	1	2	3	4	5
I would rather have people think that I am lazy than stupid	1	2	3	4	5
It is important to me to always do better than others.	1	2	3	4	5
I give up too easily when I am faced with a difficult task.	1	2	3	4	5

Appendix B

Invitation to Program

Dear Program Director:

I am writing to ask your cooperation in a research study investigating the relationship between achievement motivation and student age in physician assistant students. Currently, I am the associate director of academic affairs at Kettering College of Medical Arts Physician Assistant Program in Kettering, Ohio. I am also a doctoral student at Walden University and this study is the subject of my doctoral dissertation.

Researchers have confirmed important differences in the motivational attitudes of younger and older students that impact their motivational goals and thus their academic performance. However, few studies have investigated the relationship of achievement motivation and student age at the collegiate level and no studies have been directed at physician assistant students.

For this study, only first year, bachelor's students will be eligible to participate. Students who agree to take part in the study will be asked to complete the *Goals Inventory*, a 24 item Likert Scale questionnaire printed on a Scantron form. On this Scantron form students will also record their date of birth. This should take no more than 10-15 minutes to complete. I will provide you with all necessary materials and all you have to do is collect the instruments once students have completed them and mail it back to me in the provided self addressed envelope.

Your assistance in this research study would be greatly appreciated. Please complete the attached information form designating a site coordinator/contact person for the study and return it via e-mail. I will then contact you shortly after I receive your completed form with further information. Should you have any questions concerning this study please call me at 937-298-3399 Ext. 55607 or 513-934-4091. I appreciate your consideration and look forward to working with you.

Sincerely,

Mona Sedrak, MS, PA-C
Associate Director of Academic Affairs
Physician Assistant Studies
Kettering College Medical Arts

Appendix C

Program Informational Form

Program Name:

Program Address:

Program Telephone Number:

Name of Program Director:

Designated Site Coordinator/ Contact Person:

Number of 1st year bachelor students currently enrolled:

Please return via e-mail to: <u>msedrak@waldenu.edu</u>
Thank-you for your cooperation!

Appendix D

Instructions for Site Coordinator

Dear Site Coordinator:

Thank you for agreeing to participate in this research study. Enclosed in this packet are the following items:

1. Invitation to Participate/Consent Statement to be read to students introducing the study and inviting them to participate.
2. A copy of the Invitation to Participate/Consent Statement for each participant.
3. Survey instruments.
4. Self-addressed, postage-paid return envelope.

Instructions to Site Coordinator

1. It is preferable that students are given this questionnaire at a single sitting, similar to an exam. However, if it is more convenient, the questionnaires can be administered on an individual basis. This instrument generally takes 10-15 minutes to complete. However, students may take as long as they wish.
2. Please read the enclosed Invitation to Participate/Consent Statement to the students and give each participant a copy for their records.
3. Instruct students to complete the *Goals Inventory* using a #2 lead pencil.
4. Please, instruct students **NOT** to fill in their name anywhere on the survey instrument.
5. After students have completed the survey, ask them to place it in the provided return envelope. It is preferable that the site coordinator not collect the survey

themselves, but rather have students place it in the envelope themselves to ensure confidentiality.

6. Please mail all completed surveys to the researcher.

Appendix E

Invitation to Participate/Consent Statement

The Relationship of Achievement Motivation and Student Age In Physician Assistant Students

You are invited to participate in a research study that investigates the relationship between student age and achievement goal orientation. This study is being conducted by Mona Sedrak, MS, PA-C, a doctoral candidate at Walden University. Only first year PA students enrolled an accredited bachelor's degree awarding PA Program are eligible to participate in this study.

The purpose of this study is to help educators better understand the motivational differences that may exist between older and younger students and how these differences impact academic performance. To assess achievement goal orientation, you will be asked to complete the *Goals Inventory*, a 24-question survey instrument. All surveys are coded, therefore your identity will be protected. This instrument should take no more than 10-15 minutes of your time to complete. The only personal information you will be asked to provide is your age.

All information collected, as part of this research will be held in the strictest confidence. At no time will information regarding specific students be released to any individuals or institutions. While analysis of this information may be published in the future, at no time will your name or identifying information be used. Research records will be kept in a locked file and only the researcher will have access to the records.

Your decision whether or not to participate will not effect your current or future relations with your academic institution or Walden University. If you decide to participate, you are free to withdraw at any time without affecting those relationships. Should you choose to participate, you will be given a copy of this information to keep for your records. If you have any questions about this study, you may contact the following individuals:

Mona Sedrak, MS, PA-C
1076 Heritage Trace
Lebanon, OH, 45036
513-934-4091

Sybil Delevan, PhD
401 South 1st Street #1312
Minneapolis, MN 55401
612-333-2231

Appendix F

Permission to Use Instrument

Theresa DeBacker, PhD

Date: Tue, 25 Sep 2001 16:16:38 –0500
From: "Teresa K. DeBacker" <debacker@ou.edu>
Subject: Re: goals inventory
To: msedrak <msedrak@waldenu.edu>
X-Mailer: Mozilla 4.72 [en] (Win98; U)
X-Accept-Language: en

Mona,

You have my permission to use the goals inventory. I assume you have the 1994 article in Educational and Psychological Measurement. You can reproduce the questionnaire by putting the items listed in Table 1 into numerical order and providing a 5-point Likert scale (1 = never true of me, 5 = always true of me) for students to use when they respond.

Good luck with your study,

Teresa K. DeBacker, Ph.D.
Associate Professor and Program Coordinator
Instructional Psychology and Technology Program
University of Oklahoma

Greg Schraw, PhD

Date: Mon, 24 Sep 2001 15:50:30 -0700
From: Greg Schraw <gschraw@unlv.edu>
X-Mailer: Mozilla 4.75 [en] (Win98; U)
X-Accept-Language: en
To: msedrak <msedrak@waldenu.edu>
Subject: Re: goals inventory

Hi Mona,
 Please feel free to use the Goals Inventory. I assume you have a copy of the instrument and validation paper. If not, I will attach a copy for you.

Gregg

Mona M. Sedrak
1076 Heritage Trace
Lebanon OH 45036

EDUCATION

2000 – 2003 Doctor of Philosophy, Education / Higher Education – Walden University
1999 – 2000 Master of Science, Advanced PA Studies/ Education – A.T. Stills University/ Kirksville College of Osteopathic Medicine
1987 - 1990 Bachelor of Science, Allied Health Studies - University of Texas Southwestern Medical Center of Dallas/ Physician Assistant Program

CERTIFICATES & LICENSES

1990 – Present NCCPA certified
1999- Present Ohio Licensure

PROFESSIONAL EXPERIENCE

2000 – Present Kettering College of Medical Arts, Physician Assistant Program
Associate Director of Academic Affairs
Kettering, OH

2000- Present A.T. Stills University/ Kirksville College of Osteopathic Medicine
Master of Science/ Advanced Physician Assistant Studies
Faculty and Coordinator of the Education/ Leadership Track
Distance Education
Mesa, AZ

2003- Present Wright State University/ Department of Family Medicine
Research Associate
Dayton, OH

1999-2000 Health Alliance – Occnet
Director of Operations/ Occnet Mineola & St. Louis East Clinics
Erlanger, OH

1998 -1999 Health Partners- Occupational and Environmental Medicine
Physician Assistant/ Clinic Supervisor
St. Paul, MN

1995 – 1997 Medical and Surgical Group of Irving
Physician Assistant- Family Medicine
Irving, TX

1992- 1995	Occusystems Physician Assistant – Occupational Medicine Dallas, TX
1991 – 1992	Texas Scottish Rite Hospital Physician Assistant – Pediatric Neurology Dallas, TX

AWARDS

12-2001	Physician Assistant Faculty of the Year, Kettering College of Medical Arts.

PUBLICATIONS

Mona M. Sedrak. "Peripheral Neuropathies." In J. Labus *The Physician Assistant Handbook*. In press.

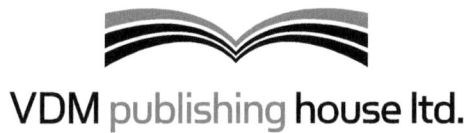

VDM publishing house ltd.

Scientific Publishing House
offers
free of charge publication
of current academic research papers, Bachelor´s Theses, Master's Theses, Dissertations or Scientific Monographs

If you have written a thesis which satisfies high content as well as formal demands, and you are interested in a remunerated publication of your work, please send an e-mail with some initial information about yourself and your work to *info@vdm-publishing-house.com.*

Our editorial office will get in touch with you shortly.

VDM Publishing House Ltd.
Meldrum Court 17.
Beau Bassin
Mauritius
www.vdm-publishing-house.com

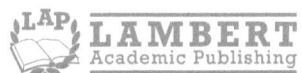
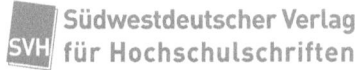

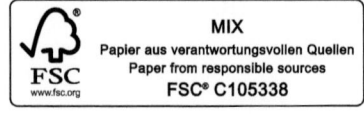

Printed by Books on Demand GmbH, Norderstedt / Germany